Metastatic Neoplasms in Fine-Needle Aspiration Cytology

Yun Gong

Metastatic Neoplasms in Fine-Needle Aspiration Cytology

Diagnostic Tips and Traps

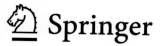 Springer

Yun Gong
Professor
Department of Pathology
The University of Texas
MD Anderson Cancer Center
Houston, TX, USA

ISBN 978-3-319-23620-9   ISBN 978-3-319-23621-6   (eBook)
DOI 10.1007/978-3-319-23621-6

Library of Congress Control Number: 2015949645

Springer Cham Heidelberg New York Dordrecht London
© Springer International Publishing Switzerland 2016
This work is subject to copyright. All rights are reserved by the Publisher, whether
the whole or part of the material is concerned, specifically the rights of translation,
reprinting, reuse of illustrations, recitation, broadcasting, reproduction on
microfilms or in any other physical way, and transmission or information storage
and retrieval, electronic adaptation, computer software, or by similar or dissimilar
methodology now known or hereafter developed.
The use of general descriptive names, registered names, trademarks, service marks,
etc. in this publication does not imply, even in the absence of a specific statement,
that such names are exempt from the relevant protective laws and regulations and
therefore free for general use.
The publisher, the authors and the editors are safe to assume that the advice and
information in this book are believed to be true and accurate at the date of
publication. Neither the publisher nor the authors or the editors give a warranty,
express or implied, with respect to the material contained herein or for any errors or
omissions that may have been made.

Printed on acid-free paper

Springer International Publishing AG Switzerland is part of Springer Science+Business
Media (www.springer.com)

To my family, colleagues, and fellows for their love and support

Preface

To effectively help a clinician make an optimal personalized therapeutic decision, it is important for a cytopathologist not only to
make an accurate diagnosis on fine-needle aspiration (FNA)
samples but also to provide prognostic and therapeutically predictive information. Knowledge of clinicians' needs and clinical
impact of a FNA diagnosis is of paramount importance during the
workup of a metastatic neoplasm.

This book provides a road map with which to navigate the
thought process in reaching a proper final FNA diagnosis. In contrast to most cytology books that describe the morphologic features
and ancillary study findings of each disease entities in various
organ systems in a "horizontal and detail manner," this book is
organized in a "longitudinal and cohesive fashion" to address diagnostic thought process, starting from rapid on-site immediate
evaluation and sample triage strategy. The main framework of
diagnostic approach includes metastatic pattern, morphologic pattern, and immunophenotypic pattern. The morphologic evaluation
is stratified into lineage-specific and lineage-nonspecific patterns
and the general cytologic features and differential diagnoses of the
major entities/subtypes (rather than each individual tumor entities)
are summarized. A systematic, tired algorithm is well outlined in
immunoperoxidase workup. The pitfalls or traps that may be
encountered in daily practice are emphasized and the solutions or
tips are provided together with high-quality cytologic images,
many of which have corresponding histologic or cell block images
and immunostaining illustrations. A multidisciplinary approach is
the key to avoid erroneous diagnosis.

This book may also serve as a reference for commonly used immunostaining makers (Tables 4.1 and 4.2) and characteristic phenotypes of the common tumor entities within each of the four major lineages (i.e., epithelial, melanocytic, hematopoietic, and mesenchymal) (Tables 4.8, 4.9, 4.10, and 4.11) and their main subtypes. Flow cytometric immunophenotyping, cytogenetic, and molecular studies including recently developed and promising markers that may change pathology practice are also covered.

In the era of molecular diagnostics and targeted personalized therapy, a high-quality tumor sample is imperative. The book shares practical experience of MD Anderson and covers the strategies regarding how to use small and limited FNA samples for making the most informative diagnosis and how to preserve tumor tissues for cytogenetic and genomic tests that, in turn, facilitate diagnosis and targeted therapies.

I believe that this book is a helpful complement to many excellent cytologic books and hope that you will find the book useful in your daily practice. Any feedback from you is very much welcomed.

Special Acknowledgment

The author wishes to express her gratitude to the following for their valuable help to the book:

Kim-Anh T Vu at the Department of Pathology for editing images of the book.

Houston, TX, USA   Yun Gong, MD

Contents

Abbreviations and Other Names of Immunomarkers

AFP   Alpha fetoprotein
ALK   Anaplastic lymphoma kinase
AMACR   Alpha-methylacyl-CoA racemase,
            also named as P504S
AR   Androgen receptor
β-HCG   Beta-human chorionic gonadotropin
BCL   B-cell lymphoma
CAIX   Carbonic anhydrase IX
CD   Cluster of differentiation
CD15   Also named as LeuM1
CD30   Also named as Ki-1
CD45   Also named as LCA (leukocyte common
            antigen)
CD68   Also named as KP1
CD99   Also named as MIC2
CD117   Also named as cKit
CDH17   Cadherin-17
CDK4   Cyclin-dependent kinase 4
CDX2   Caudal type homeobox 2
CEA   Carcinoembryonic antigen
CK   Cytokeratin
CK903   Also named as 34βE12
D2-40   Also named as podoplanin
DOG1   Discovered on GIST-1
EMA   Epithelial membrane antigen
ER   Estrogen receptor
ERG   ETS-related gene
FLI1   Friend leukemia virus integration 1

GATA3	GATA binding protein 3
GCDFP	Gross cystic disease fluid protein, also named as BRST2
INI1	Integrase interactor 1
HepPar1	Hepatocyte paraffin-1
HMB45	Human melanoma black 45
HPV	Human papillomavirus
Ki67	Also named as MIB-1 (mindbomb homolog 1)
MART1	Melanoma-associated antigen recognized by T-cells 1
MCPyV	Merkel cell polyomavirus
MDM2	Mouse double minute 2 homolog
MITF	Microphthalmia-associated transcription factor
MPO	Myeloperoxidase
MSA	Muscle-specific actin
MUM1	Multiple myeloma 1, also named as IRF4 (interferon regulatory factor 4)
MyoD1	Myogenic differentiation 1
NANOG	NANOG homeobox
NKX2.2	NK2 homeobox 2
NKX3.1	NK3 homeobox 1
NY-ESO-1	New York esophageal squamous cell carcinoma 1
OCT3/4	Octamer-binding transcription factor 3/4
PanCK	Pancytokeratin
PAX	Paired box gene
PR	Progesterone receptor
PAP	Prostate-specific acid phosphatase, also named as PSAP
PLAP	Placental alkaline phosphatase
Prostein	Also named as P501S
PSA	Prostate-specific antigen
PTH	Parathyroid hormone
RCC	Renal cell carcinoma marker
Sall4	Sal-like protein 4
SATB2	Special AT-rich sequence-binding protein 2
STAT6	Single transducers and activators of transcription 6

SF1	Steroidogenic factor 1
SMA	Smooth muscle actin
SOX	Sex-determining region Y box
TdT	Terminal deoxytransferase
TFE3	Transcription factor binding to IGHM enhancer 3
TLE1	Transducin-like enhancer of split 1
TTF1	Thyroid transcription factor 1
WT1	Wilms tumor 1

Chapter 1
Introduction

Fine-needle aspiration (FNA) is a safe, simple, rapid, and cost-effective procedure that allows the acquisition of samples not only from superficial and large lesions but also from small or deep-seated lesions. In addition, it allows for sampling multiple lesions during the same biopsy procedure. Therefore, FNA is often used as an initial diagnostic modality to work up metastatic tumors at almost any body site. It provides valuable information that enables clinicians and oncologists to evaluate patients' prognosis and design optimal therapeutic strategies, including planning preoperative management for patients with operable tumors and choosing adequate medical therapy for patients with non-resectable tumors or hematopoietic malignancies.

To make a proper cytologic diagnosis, these key questions should be considered step by step:

- Is the lesion neoplastic or nonneoplastic?
- If it is neoplastic, is it benign or malignant?
- If it is malignant, what is its cell lineage (i.e., epithelial, melanocytic, hematopoietic, or mesenchymal)?
- In cases of epithelial malignancy (i.e., carcinoma), what is the subtype (e.g., adenocarcinoma, squamous carcinoma, neuroendocrine carcinoma, or others)?
- If it is a malignant tumor, is it a primary tumor or a metastatic disease (regardless of its cell lineage)?
- If it is a metastasis, what is its primary origin?

© Springer International Publishing Switzerland 2016
Y. Gong, *Metastatic Neoplasms in Fine-Needle Aspiration Cytology*, DOI 10.1007/978-3-319-23621-6_1

The main strategies used in an FNA diagnosis of metastatic malignancies are as follows:

- Identifying cells that are "foreign" to the aspiration site to ensure a metastatic nature
- Correlating FNA findings with a clinical history (i.e., previous malignancy and current presentation) and radiologic findings
- Knowledge of the general metastatic pattern and morphologic pattern of various tumors
- Using ancillary studies if necessary
- Reviewing previous cytologic or surgical pathologic material and comparing morphologic features with those of the current lesion
- Consulting experts if necessary
- For insolvable cases, recommending tissue biopsy for histologic confirmation

This book provides a road map with which to navigate the thought process in reaching a proper final FNA diagnosis, with an emphasis on tumors in the metastatic setting. An algorithmic approach to FNA diagnosis (including the metastatic pattern, morphologic pattern, and immunophenotypic pattern) is outlined in Fig. 1.1 and will be expanded in subsequent chapters. Sample collection, triage, and recommendations for ancillary studies and molecular studies are covered as well.

Metastatic Pattern

Metastasis is one of the complicated biological properties of tumor cells. Usually, metastasis occurs in an orderly sequence: local invasion, breakthrough of the basement membrane, intravasation and survival in the blood or lymph stream, extravasation, colonization, and proliferation. Most metastases follow a predictable route of dissemination on the bases of the circulatory map. Locoregional metastasis usually occurs first, with a pattern corresponding to the blood or lymphatic drainage of the primary neoplasm; distant metastasis usually occurs later. The common destinations of distant metastases are the vascular organs, such as the liver, lungs,

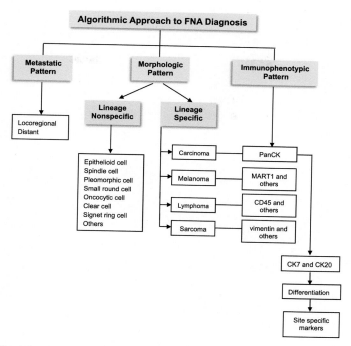

Fig. 1.1 Algorithmic approach to fine-needle aspiration cytology diagnosis of metastatic tumors

and brain. Bone is another preferential target of distant metastasis, although it is not a particularly vascular site. Notably, metastasis occurs more frequently in these organ sites than do primary tumors, and sometimes, metastatic tumors can cytologically resemble primary tumors of these sites. For example, adenocarcinoma of the pancreaticobiliary tract in the lungs often shows a bronchioloalveolar or "airway" growth pattern, mimicking primary bronchioloalveolar carcinoma of the lungs (Fig. 1.2).

In general, carcinomas tend to metastasize via the lymphatics and initially involve the lymph nodes, whereas sarcomas tend to metastasize hematogenously to visceral organs such as the liver and lungs. However, for gastrointestinal epithelial malignancies, the liver is the most common recipient due to the characteristic

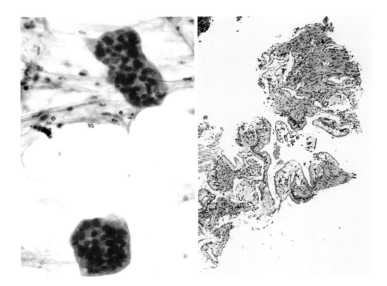

Fig. 1.2 Metastatic pancreatic adenocarcinoma to the lung often shows "airway" growth pattern, resembling a primary mucinous bronchioloalveolar carcinoma (*left*, Papanicolaou stain; *right*, H&E-stained cell block)

anatomic venous pathway. The common metastatic pattern of various tumors and the common primary origins of various metastatic sites are listed in decreasing frequency, on the basis of published studies, in Tables 1.1 and 1.2. Familiarity with the common metastatic pattern helps to predict the location of the primary tumor during the workup of FNA cases.

However, exception is not uncommon. Some tumors have a preferential distribution of metastasis that is not explainable by the natural pathways of drainage. For example, renal cell carcinoma and follicular thyroid carcinoma tend to disseminate hematogenously. Lobular breast carcinoma has a tendency to spread to the abdominal cavity, especially to the gastrointestinal tract, ovaries, and serosal surfaces. Likewise, while most sarcomas rarely metastasize to the lymph nodes, some sarcomas tend to involve lymph nodes, such as synovial sarcoma, angiosarcoma, rhabdomyosarcoma, epithelioid sarcoma, follicular dendritic cell sarcoma, and

Table 1.1 Common metastatic sites of various malignancies

Primary origin of malignant tumor	Lymph node metastasis	Distant metastasis
Carcinoma		
Adrenal gland	Regional LNs	Liver, lung, bone
Anorectal site	Inguinal, mesenteric LNs	Liver, lung
Bladder	Pelvic, iliac, obturator, sacral, retroperitoneal LNs	Lung, liver, bone
Breast	Axillary, internal mammary, supraclavicular, infraclavicular LNs	Bone, lung, liver, brain, adrenal gland, pleura (lobular CA may metastasize to GI and GYN sites, endocrine organs)
Cervix	Pelvic, inguinal, retroperitoneal LNs	Lung, bowel
Colorectal site	Regional LNs	Liver, lung, peritoneum
Head and neck	Regional LNs, parotid gland	
Esophagus	Regional LNs, supraclavicular LN	Liver, lung, peritoneum
Kidney	LN metastasis is rare. Regional LNs	Lung, bone, liver, adrenal gland, brain, unusual sites (thyroid, small bone, others)
Liver, hepatocellular CA	Regional LNs	Liver, lung, bone, adrenal gland
Liver, cholangiocarcinoma	Regional LNs	Lung, bone, adrenal gland, peritoneum
Lung	Hilar, mediastinal, supraclavicular LNs	Lung, adrenal gland, liver, bone, pleura, brain
Ovary	Iliac, obturator, inguinal, pelvic, retroperitoneal LNs	Peritoneum, pleura, lung
Pancreas	Regional LNs	Liver, peritoneum, lung (may mimic mucinous BAC)

(continued)

Table 1.1 (continued)

Primary origin of malignant tumor	Lymph node metastasis	Distant metastasis
Parathyroid	Regional LNs	Lung, liver, bone
Prostate	Pelvic, obturator, iliac, sacral, retroperitoneal, supraclavicular LNs	Bone (spine, femur, pelvis, rib), lung, liver, adrenal gland
Gonadal or extragonadal sites (germ cell tumors)	Mediastinal LN, retroperitoneal LNs, supraclavicular LN	Lung (most common), liver brain, bone
Thyroid	Regional LNs (usually for papillary and medullary CA)	Lung, bone, liver (for follicular and medullary CA)
Salivary gland	Regional LNs, neck LNs	Lung
Stomach	Regional LNs, left supraclavicular (Virchow) LN, periumbilical node (Sister Mary Joseph nodule)	Peritoneum, liver, ovary (Krukenberg tumor)
Uterus	Pelvic, retroperitoneal LNs	Lung, peritoneum, vagina
Melanoma	Regional LNs, distant LNs	Lung, liver, skin, soft tissue, adrenal gland, brain; intraocular melanoma exclusively metastasizes to liver
Sarcoma	LN metastasis is rare	Lung (most common), liver, bone
Lymphoma	Superficial LNs, abdominal LNs, pelvic LNs, and retroperitoneal LNs	Various extranodal organ sites

Abbreviations: *BAC* bronchioloalveolar carcinoma, *CA* carcinoma, *GI* gastrointestinal, *GYN* gynecologic, *LN* lymph node

Kaposi sarcoma. Furthermore, some tumors have a more restricted range of target tissues than others: ocular melanoma is almost exclusively confined to the liver, whereas melanoma of elsewhere can metastasize to virtually every organ site. The unpredictable

Table 1.2 Common primary origins of various metastatic sites

Metastatic site	Common primary origin of malignant tumor
Cervical LNs	Thyroid, salivary gland, other head and neck sites, melanoma, lung, esophagus
Intraparotid LNs	Head and neck squamous carcinoma, melanoma, salivary gland
Axillary LNs	Breast
Supraclavicular LNs	Breast, lung, stomach, esophagus, lymphoma
Hilar/mediastinal LNs	Lung, breast, germ cell tumors, lymphoma
Abdominal LNs	Colon, rectum, stomach, esophagus, pancreaticobiliary tract, uterus, ovary, lymphoma
Pelvic LNs	Prostate, ovary, uterus, bladder
Inguinal LNs	Anorectal, vulva, vagina, uterine cervix, penis, scrotum, melanoma
Retroperitoneal LNs	Kidney, colon, prostate, uterus, ovary
Adrenal gland	Lung, kidney, breast, thyroid
Bone	Breast, prostate, lung, kidney, thyroid
Brain	Lung, breast, kidney, colon, melanoma, thyroid, liver
Cerebrospinal fluid	Breast, melanoma, lymphoma, acute leukemia
Kidney	Lung, breast, colon, melanoma
Heart	Lung, breast
Liver	Colon, rectum, pancreas, stomach, esophagus, breast, lung, kidney, melanoma, sarcoma
Lung	Breast, lung, colon, kidney, melanoma, prostate, sarcoma, germ cell tumors
Pancreas	Lung, breast, kidney
Peritoneum	Ovary, colon, rectum, stomach, esophagus, pancreaticobiliary tract, uterus
Pleura	Lung, breast
Salivary gland	Head and neck squamous carcinoma, melanoma
Thyroid	Kidney, lung, breast, colon, melanoma

Abbreviation: *LN* lymph node

pattern of metastasis may pose a diagnostic difficulty for clinicians and pathologists and may result in an erroneous diagnosis. Figures 1.3, 1.4, 1.5, 1.6, 1.7, and 1.8 illustrate examples of unusual metastatic patterns.

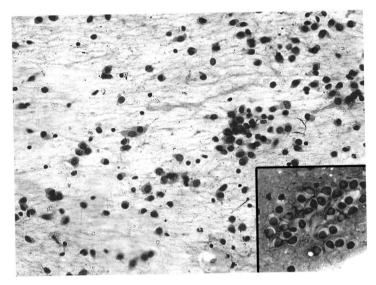

Fig. 1.3 Unusual metastatic pattern (example 1): metastatic myxoid chondrosarcoma in an inguinal lymph node (Papanicolaou stain; *inset*, Diff-Quik stain)

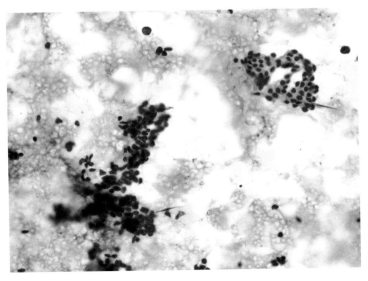

Fig. 1.4 Unusual metastatic pattern (example 2): metastatic small cell carcinoma of the lung to a colloid nodule in the thyroid. The cells in the right upper corner are benign thyroid follicular cells (Papanicolaou stain)

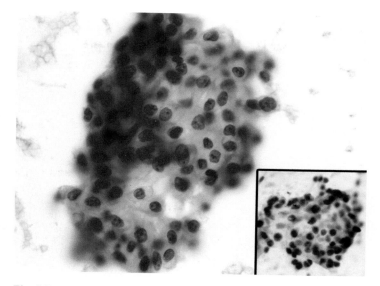

Fig. 1.5 Unusual metastatic pattern (example 3): metastatic renal cell carcinoma (clear cell type) in soft tissue of the skull and verified by positive PAX8 staining on a smear (Papanicolaou stain; *inset*, PAX8 stain)

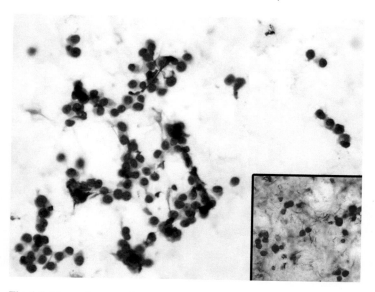

Fig. 1.6 Unusual metastatic pattern (example 4): metastatic melanoma in the breast with plasmacytoid appearance, resembling cytologic features of lobular breast carcinoma. The diagnosis was confirmed by positive MART1 staining on a smear (Papanicolaou stain; *inset*, MART1 stain)

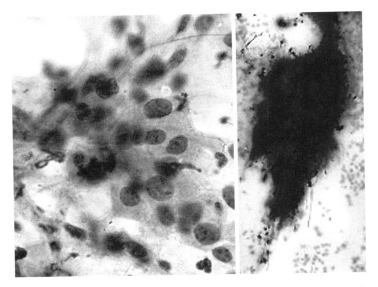

Fig. 1.7 Unusual metastatic pattern (example 5): metaplastic breast carcinoma with myxochondroid matrix in the thyroid (*left*, Papanicolaou stain; *right*, Diff-Quik stain)

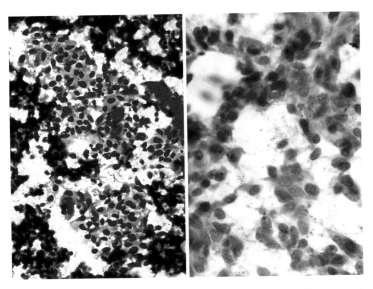

Fig. 1.8 Unusual metastatic pattern (example 6): metastatic papillary thyroid carcinoma in soft tissue of the thigh (*left*, Diff-Quik stain; *right*, Papanicolaou stain)

Morphologic Pattern

The morphologic patterns of different tumors can be categorized into lineage-specific patterns and lineage-nonspecific patterns (Fig. 1.1). Tumors in lineage-specific patterns are derived from one of the four major lineages (the "Big 4"): epithelial (i.e., carcinoma), melanocytic (i.e., melanoma), hematopoietic (mostly lymphoma but also plasma cell neoplasms and myeloid sarcoma), and mesenchymal (i.e., sarcoma). Figure 1.9 outlines the tumors of

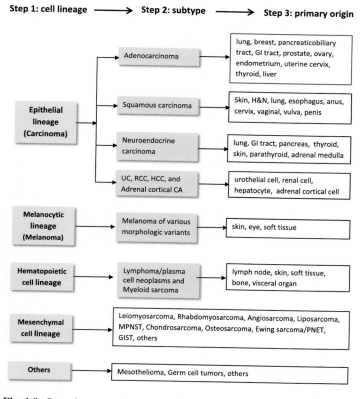

Fig. 1.9 Stepwise approach to fine-needle aspiration diagnosis of metastatic tumors: lineage, subtype, and primary site determination Abbreviations: *CA* carcinoma, *GI* gastrointestinal, *GIST* gastrointerstinal stromal tumor, *HCC* hepatocellular carcinoma, *H&N* head and neck, *MPNST* malignant peripheral nerve sheath tumor, *PNET* primitive neuroectodermal tumor, *RCC* renal cell carcinoma, *UC* urothelial carcinoma

various lineages, their subtypes, and their common primary origins. FNA diagnosis should follow the algorithm step by step.

In contrast, tumors of a lineage-nonspecific pattern have a different histogenesis but similar cytologic features. The common cytologic patterns include epithelioid cell, spindle cell, pleomorphic cell, small round cell, oncocytic cell, clear cell, and signet ring cell morphologic features (Fig. 1.10). For example, malignant tumors with epithelioid morphologic features are most commonly seen in carcinoma but can also be seen in sarcoma, melanoma, and lymphoma or plasma cell neoplasms. Likewise, malignant tumors with spindle cell features are most likely to be sarcoma but can also be spindle cell carcinoma, melanoma, and occasionally hematopoietic malignancies. The general cytologic features of each pattern will be covered in Chaps. 2 and 3.

Immunophenotypic Pattern

In routine cytology practice, diagnostic challenges are often encountered, especially when metastatic tumors appear in an unexpected site or show a lineage-nonspecific pattern or when metastasis occurs years or decades after treatment of the primary tumor. Some tumors can present as metastatic disease with an unknown primary. Even among tumors with a known lineage, such as carcinoma, tumors that are well to moderately differentiated may demonstrate distinct morphologic features suggestive of a particular subtype or even its primary origin, whereas tumors with a poorly differentiated nature may not demonstrate such specific features. Therefore, ancillary studies, especially immunoperoxidase studies, are often needed. In addition, prognostic and therapeutic markers are often tested on cytology samples for clinicians to determine the appropriate management of some tumors.

In light of the limited sample size of FNA material, which is an intrinsic problem with aspirated material, immunoperoxidase staining should be applied in a stepwise fashion. An immunoperoxidase workup of a poorly differentiated tumor or metastasis with an unknown primary often starts with cell lineage

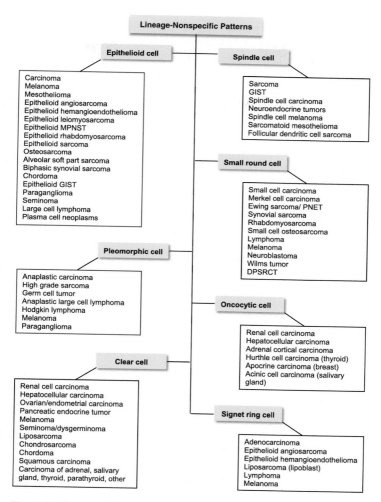

Fig. 1.10 Tumors with lineage-nonspecific patterns showing similar cytologic features but have different cell lineage or histogenesis. Abbreviations: *DPSRCT* desmoplastic small round cell tumor, *GIST* gastrointestinal stromal tumor, *MPNST* malignant peripheral nerve sheath tumor, *PNET* primitive neuroectodermal tumor

determination using one or a few first-line markers: pancytokeratin (panCK), melanocytic markers (such as MART1), and pan-hematopoietic markers (such as leukocyte common antigen, also called CD45) (Fig. 1.1).

In general, epithelial malignancy (i.e., carcinoma) accounts for the majority of malignancies and adenocarcinoma constitutes the majority of carcinomas. Further subtyping of an adenocarcinoma and identifying its primary origin often require a panel of cytokeratin 7 (CK7) and CK20 markers. However, this panel is insufficient for pinpointing a primary site in most cases, except for colorectal adenocarcinoma. Thus, the next step is to use site-specific markers, such as TTF1 for lung or thyroid origins and GATA3 for breast or urothelial origins. Of note, none of the markers are 100 % specific; thus, a panel approach and careful interpretation should be used in the context of the morphologic, clinical, and radiologic findings. A single marker might be used in a confirmatory setting when material for staining is limited. The immunophenotypic patterns of different tumors and common markers are addressed in detail in Chap. 4.

Suggested Readings

1. Abbruzzese JL, Abbruzzese MC, Lenzi R, Hess KR, Raber MN. Analysis of a diagnostic strategy for patients with suspected tumors of unknown origin. J Clin Oncol. 1995;13:2094–103.
2. Alvarez RH, Gong Y, Ueno NT, Alizadeh PA, Hortobagyi GN, Valero V. Metastasis in the breast mimicking inflammatory breast cancer. J Clin Oncol. 2012;30:e202–6.
3. Chu P, Wu E, Weiss LM. Cytokeratin 7 and cytokeratin 20 expression in epithelial neoplasms: a survey of 435 cases. Mod Pathol. 2000;13:962–72.
4. Chu PG, Weiss LM. Keratin expression in human tissues and neoplasms. Histopathology. 2002;40:403–39.
5. Disibio G, French SW. Metastatic patterns of cancers: results from a large autopsy study. Arch Pathol Lab Med. 2008;132:931–9.
6. Elsheikh TM, Herzberg AJ, Silverman JF. Fine-needle aspiration cytology of metastatic malignancies involving unusual sites. Am J Clin Pathol. 1997;108:S12–21.
7. Elsheikh TM, Silverman JF. Fine needle aspiration cytology of metastasis to common and unusual sites. Pathol Case Rev. 2001;6:161–72.

8. Gong Y. Ancillary studies on neoplastic cytologic specimens. In: Nayar R, editor. Cytology in oncology. New York: Springer; 2013. p. 13–29.

9. Gong Y, Jalali M, Staerkel G. Fine needle aspiration cytology of a thyroid metastasis of metaplastic breast carcinoma: a case report. Acta Cytol. 2005;49:327–30.

10. Hess KR, Varadhachary GR, Taylor SH, Wei W, Raber MN, Lenzi R, Abbruzzese JL. Metastatic patterns in adenocarcinoma. Cancer. 2006; 106:1624–33.

11. Leong SP, Cady B, Jablons DM, Garcia-Aguilar J, Reintgen D, Jakub J, Pendas S, Duhaime L, Cassell R, Gardner M, Giuliano R, Archie V, Calvin D, Mensha L, Shivers S, Cox C, Werner JA, Kitagawa Y, Kitajima M. Clinical patterns of metastasis. Cancer Metastasis Rev. 2006;25:221–32.

12. Lin F, Liu H. Unknown primary/undifferentiated neoplasms in surgical and cytologic specimens. In: Lin F, Prichard JW, Liu H, Wilkerson M, Schuerch C, editors. Handbook of practical immunohistochemistry: frequently asked questions. New York: Springer; 2011. p. 55–83.

13. Moll R, Franke WW, Schiller DL, Geiger B, Krepler R. The catalog of human cytokeratins: patterns of expression in normal epithelia, tumors and cultured cells. Cell. 1982;31:11–24.

14. Nguyen DX, Bos PD, Massague J. Metastasis: from dissemination to organ-specific colonization. Nat Rev Cancer. 2009;9:274–84.

15. Taylor C, Cote R. Immunomicroscopy: a diagnostic tool for the surgical pathologist, Major problems in pathology. Philadelphia: Saunders Elsevier; 2006.

16. Uzquiano MC, Prieto VG, Nash JW, Ivan DS, Gong Y, Lazar AJ, Diwan AH. Metastatic basal cell carcinoma exhibits reduced actin expression. Mod Pathol. 2008;21:540–3.

17. Wang J, Gong Y. Metastatic papillary thyroid carcinoma in the thigh with unusual cytologic features. Diagn Cytopathol. 2014;42:278–9.

18. Zhang S, Gong Y. From cytomorphology to molecular pathology: maximizing the value of cytology of lymphoproliferative disorders and soft tissue tumors. Am J Clin Pathol. 2013;140:454–67.

Chapter 2
Sample Collection, Preparation, Rapid On-Site Evaluation, and Triage

Sample Collection and Preparation

The success of an FNA procedure depends on the nature of the lesion (e.g., size, location, and consistency), the skill of the aspirator, and the availability of rapid on-site evaluation. Large palpable lesions can be aspirated by a pathologist, and small deeply seated lesions are usually aspirated by the radiologist under image guidance. Usually, a 22- to 25-gauge needle is used, and two to three needle passes are made. Aspirated materials are expressed onto several glass slides and smeared out.

Two types of stains are typically performed: Diff-Quik staining using air-dried smears and Papanicolaou staining using smears fixed in 95 % ethanol or Carnoy's solution. Both stains are complementary for cytologic diagnosis. Diff-Quik staining preferably highlights cytoplasmic details and extracellular or background contents, whereas Papanicolaou staining allows better visualization of nuclear characteristics such as the nuclear membrane, chromatin, and nucleoli. In some laboratories, liquid-based preparations (e.g., ThinPrep and SurePath) may be used.

Cells retained in the needle hub are rinsed into cell-preservative medium (e.g., RPMI-1640 medium) and usually spun down to make cell block or cytospin slides, depending on the size of the pellet after centrifugation. However, if a hematopoietic malignancy is suspected on the basis of clinical or cytologic findings and a flow cytometric immunophenotyping is anticipated, fresh cells should be preferentially collected and suspended in cell-preservative medium containing fetal bovine serum.

© Springer International Publishing Switzerland 2016
Y. Gong, *Metastatic Neoplasms in Fine-Needle
Aspiration Cytology*, DOI 10.1007/978-3-319-23621-6_2

Rapid On-Site Evaluation and Sample Triage

Rapid on-site evaluation ensures high diagnostic accuracy by assessing sample adequacy and determining triage strategy. It is usually performed by an on-site pathologist who correlates the cytologic findings of direct smears (Diff-Quik-stained smears, with or without Papanicolaou-stained smears) with the clinical and radiologic findings (so-called triple test).

Key factors to determine during on-site rapid evaluation in step-wise fashion:

- Neoplastic vs. nonneoplastic
- Benign vs. malignant if neoplastic
- Cell lineage of the tumor
- Subtype of the tumor
- Primary vs. metastatic
- Primary origin

During the triple test, detailed clinical and radiologic information should be obtained via chart review and communication with caregivers. In addition to the age, sex, clinical history, and current presentation of the patient, it is important to obtain radiologic information about the current lesion. For example, for a pulmonary lesion, it is helpful to know the size, location (central vs. peripheral and upper lobe vs. lower lobe), number (solitary vs. multiple), margin (well circumscribed vs. poorly defined), and other information (such as the presence of a cavitary component or hilar lymphadenopathy and a history of smoking). The presence of hilar lymphadenopathy and a smoking history favor a primary lung carcinoma over metastasis. For a patient with a history of breast carcinoma, it is helpful to know the primary cancer type (ductal, lobular, or others), the histologic and nuclear grade, the lymph node status and hormone receptor status, and the interval duration from the primary cancer diagnosis to the current FNA and location of the new lesion (locoregional vs. distant site). Abnormal laboratory (serum) findings may also provide useful diagnostic clue of some tumors, for example, CA19.9 in pancreatic adenocarcinoma, AFP in hepatocellular carcinoma and some germ cell tumors, CA125 in ovarian serous carcinoma, calcitonin in medullary thyroid carcinoma, and PSA in prostatic adenocarcinoma. Common conditions should be considered first before considering rare scenarios.

Sample adequacy is determined on the basis of a triple test. If a sample contains material representative of the target lesion found in clinical or radiologic assessment, the sample is considered "adequate." If a sample is scant in cellularity or contains fibrotic tissue that is incompatible with the clinical or radiologic findings or shows significant cellular distortion or artifacts, it is deemed to be "inadequate." In any case with a mismatched triple test, additional material should be requested.

Any FNA sample that appears to be adequate during on-site evaluation should be triaged properly to ensure that a definitive yet informative diagnosis can be rendered. The strategy of sample triage relies on the cytologic features of the direct smears during rapid on-site evaluation using low and high magnification (Table 2.1). The general features of malignancy are listed in Table 2.2. Sample triage may need to request additional aspirates for making a cell block which allows for better architectural assessment and potential immunostaining, for microorganism

Table 2.1 Cytologic evaluation

Low magnification
Cellularity (high, moderate, low)
Cell arrangement (cohesive, dyshesive, papillary, ductal, acinar, isolated cells)
Cell shape (epithelioid, spindle, small round cell, pleomorphic cell)
Background/extracellular contents (mucin; myxoid, chondroid, colloid, and amyloid material; hyaline globules; lymphoglandular bodies; inflammatory or necrotic debris)
High magnification
Cell border (distinct vs. indistinct)
Cytoplasmic features (amount, granularity, pigments, mucin droplet, vacuoles, perinuclear hof in plasma cells, and dark blue cytoplasmic membrane in lymphoid lesions)
Nuclear/cytoplasmic (N/C) ratio
Nuclear features (pleomorphism, chromatin pattern, nuclear membrane, inclusion, nucleolus, mitotic figure)

Table 2.2 General cytologic features of malignancy

Cellularity: increased
Cell arrangement: haphazard, three-dimensional, crowded groups, flat sheets with nuclear disorientation, discohesive clusters or numerous isolated cells
Cytoplasm: scant or variable amount with increased N/C ratio
Nuclear feature: enlarged, anisonucleosis, irregular nuclear membrane, abnormal chromatin, prominent nucleoli, mitotic figures (especially atypical forms)
Background: necrotic

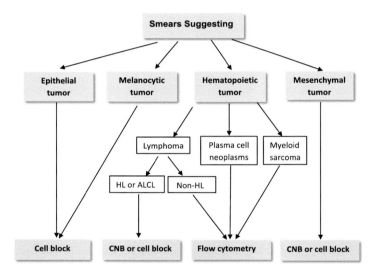

Fig. 2.1 Strategy to triage fine needle aspiration samples during rapid on-site evaluation. Abbreviations: *ALCL* anaplastic large cell lymphoma, *CNB* core needle biopsy, *HL* Hodgkin lymphoma, *Non-HL* non-Hodgkin lymphoma

cultures if the lesion appears to be infectious in nature, for flow cytometric immunophenotyping if non-Hodgkin lymphoma is suspected, for cytogenetic and molecular studies if small blue cell tumor in pediatric patients is encountered, or targeted therapy is possibly applied and for requesting a concurrent core needle biopsy if sarcoma or Hodgkin lymphoma is suspected (Fig. 2.1). Cytologic features on smears that are suggestive of each of the "Big 4" categories are summarized below.

General Features of Carcinoma (Fig. 2.2)

- Variable cellularity
- Epithelioid atypical cells
- Cohesive or syncytial groups, loosely cohesive or isolated cells (depending on tumor subtype and differentiation)
- Well-defined cell borders and a variable amount of cytoplasm
- Showing morphologic clues of specific subtypes (e.g., adenocarcinoma, squamous carcinoma, neuroendocrine carcinoma, urothelial carcinoma, renal cell carcinoma, hepatocellular carcinoma, and adrenal cortical carcinoma) (see section "Lineage-Specific Pattern" in Chap. 3 and Fig. 1.9)
- Differential diagnosis: different subtypes of carcinoma and non-epithelial tumors with an epithelioid appearance (see section "Lineage-Nonspecific Pattern" in Chap. 3 and Fig. 1.10)

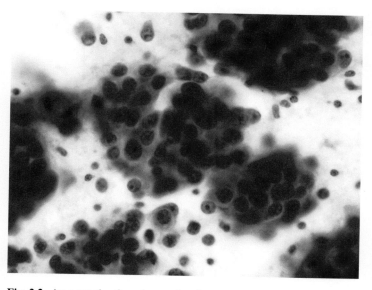

Fig. 2.2 An example of carcinoma showing atypical epithelioid cells forming cohesive groups and occasional loosely cohesive or isolated cells (Papanicolaou stain)

General Features of Melanoma (Fig. 2.3)

- High cellularity
- Epithelioid appearance with loose cohesive, discohesive, or single cells (spindle cell variant tends to be more cohesive)
- Plasmacytoid cells with eccentric nuclei and occasional binucleated or multinucleated cells. Several variants (e.g., spindle cell, small cell, and clear cell types) may be seen, as a sole type or in combination with the epithelioid type.
- Cytoplasm contains small vacuoles, with or without melanin pigment
- Dispersed chromatin and prominent nucleoli (macronucleoli) and intranuclear pseudo-inclusions
- Differential diagnosis: melanoma can resemble a wide variety of tumors with different lineages and different origins ("great mimicker")

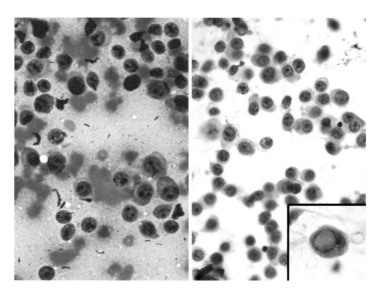

Fig. 2.3 An example of epithelioid melanoma showing plasmacytoid cells and occasional binucleated cells arranged in discohesive or single cell pattern; macronucleoli and intranuclear pseudo-inclusions are characteristic (*left*, Diff-Quik stain; *right* and *inset*, Papanicolaou stain)

General Features of Hematopoietic Neoplasms

Features of Lymphoid Cells (Fig. 2.4)

- Discohesive or single cell pattern
- Scant cytoplasm with high nuclear/cytoplasmic (N/C) ratio
- Dark blue cytoplasmic membrane (readily seen in Diff-Quik stain)
- Usually coarse chromatin (better seen in Papanicolaou stain)
- Lymphoglandular bodies (i.e., detached cytoplasmic fragments) in the background (better seen in Diff-Quik stain)

Non-Hodgkin Lymphoma (Fig. 2.5)

- Monomorphous or a mixture of small to large lymphoid cells (depending on subtype)
- Atypical small-, intermediate-, or large-sized lymphoid cells

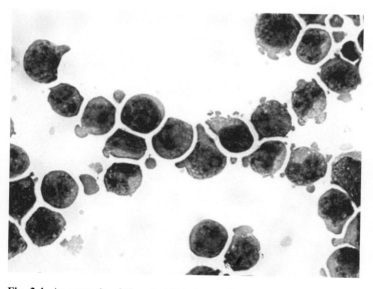

Fig. 2.4 An example of "lymphoid" lesion: cells with scant cytoplasm and high nuclear/cytoplasmic ratio arranged in discohesive or single cell pattern; dark blue cytoplasmic membrane, coarse chromatin, and lymphoglandular bodies in the background (Diff-Quik stained cytospin)

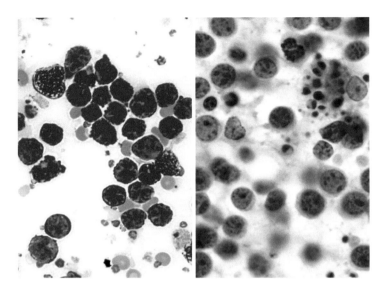

Fig. 2.5 An example of non-Hodgkin lymphoma: large B-cell lymphoma showing atypical lymphoid cells with nuclear enlargement, irregularity, prominent nucleoli, frequent mitotic figures, and apoptotic bodies (*left*, Diff-Quik stain; *right*, Papanicolaou stain)

- Abnormal chromatin (depending on maturation)
- May have nuclear irregularity and prominent nucleoli
- Differential diagnosis: reactive lymphoid hyperplasia and small round blue cell tumors (see Chap. 4)

Classical Hodgkin Lymphoma (Fig. 2.6)

- Scattered large binucleated Reed–Sternberg cells or mononucleated Hodgkin cells
- Mixed population of reactive small lymphocytes, plasma cells, eosinophils, and neutrophils in the background
- Differential diagnosis: anaplastic large cell lymphoma, large B-cell lymphoma, nodular lymphocyte-predominant Hodgkin lymphoma (see Chap. 4)

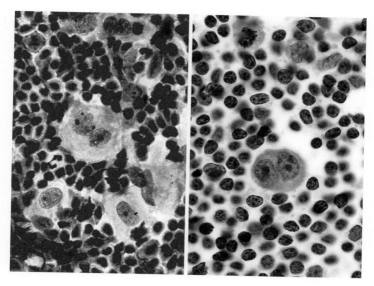

Fig. 2.6 An example of classical Hodgkin lymphoma showing scattered large binucleated Reed–Sternberg cells and mononucleated variant in a background of mixed inflammatory cells (*left*, Diff-Quik stain; *right*, Papanicolaou stain)

Plasma Cell Neoplasms (Fig. 2.7)

- Oval-shaped cells with eccentrically placed nuclei and occasional binucleated cells
- Abundant cytoplasm with paranuclear clear zone (hof) and dark blue cytoplasmic membrane (readily seen in Diff-Quik stain)
- Clumped "clockface" chromatin with indistinct nucleoli (less mature cells showing loose reticular chromatin with prominent nucleoli)
- Differential diagnosis: various tumors with plasmacytoid appearance and large cell lymphoma (Table 2.3, Figs. 1.6, 2.8, 2.9, and 2.10)

Myeloid Sarcoma (Fig. 2.11)

- Discohesive or single cell pattern
- Immature myeloid cells and myeloblasts

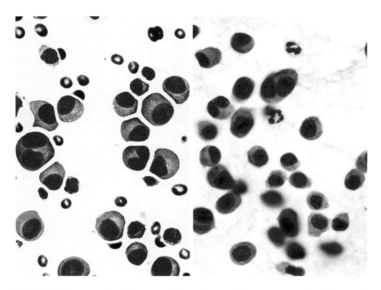

Fig. 2.7 An example of plasma cell neoplasms: plasmacytoma showing oval-shaped cells (occasional binucleated cells) with coarse, eccentric nucleus, voluminous cytoplasm with paranuclear hof, and dark blue cytoplasmic membrane (*left*, Diff-Quik stain; *right*, Papanicolaou stain)

Table 2.3 Epithelioid tumors with plasmacytoid features other than plasma cell neoplasms

Low-grade neuroendocrine carcinoma
Melanoma
Breast lobular carcinoma
Urothelial carcinoma
Medullary thyroid carcinoma
Hurthle cell tumor of the thyroid
Oncocytic or apocrine tumors
Epithelioid angiosarcoma
Rhabdomyosarcoma
Osteosarcoma
Large cell lymphoma

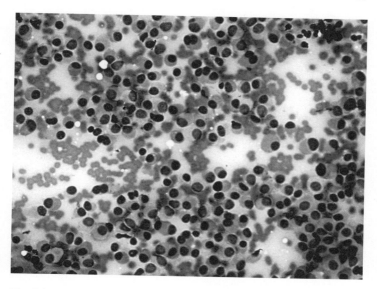

Fig. 2.8 Metastatic lobular breast carcinoma with plasmacytoid features. It should be included in the differential diagnosis of tumors with plasmacytoid appearance (Diff-Quik stain)

- Myeloblasts: large cells, moderate amount of cytoplasm, round or irregular nuclear contour, fine chromatin, and prominent nucleoli
- Differential diagnosis: lymphoma, plasma cell neoplasms, and small round blue cell tumors

General Features of Sarcoma (Fig. 2.12)

- Variably cellular
- Cohesive or dispersed single cell pattern
- Atypical pleomorphic or spindle cells, occasionally epithelioid or small round cell appearance
- Differential diagnosis: malignant tumor with spindle cell features (see section "Lineage-Nonspecific Pattern" in Chap. 3 and Fig. 1.10), benign spindle cell tumors with ancient changes such as ancient schwannoma (Fig. 2.13), nonneoplastic spindle cell proliferation such as nodular fasciitis (Fig. 2.14), and inflammatory pseudotumor

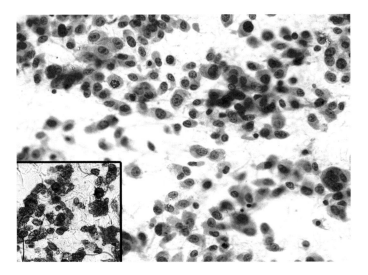

Fig. 2.9 Metastatic melanoma in the thyroid with plasmacytoid features, raising a differential diagnosis of medullary thyroid carcinoma and Hurthle cell thyroid carcinoma. The diagnosis was confirmed by positive HMB45 on a smear (Papanicolaou stain; *inset*, HMB45 stain)

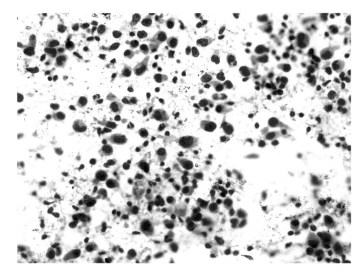

Fig. 2.10 Large B-cell lymphoma may show plasmacytoid morphology (Papanicolaou stain)

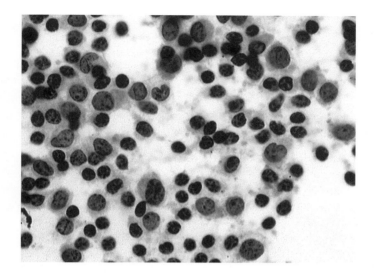

Fig. 2.11 An example of myeloid sarcoma: immature myeloid cells and myeloblasts with discohesive or single cell pattern, moderate amount of pale cytoplasm, round to kidney-shaped nuclei, fine chromatin, and prominent nucleoli (Papanicolaou stain)

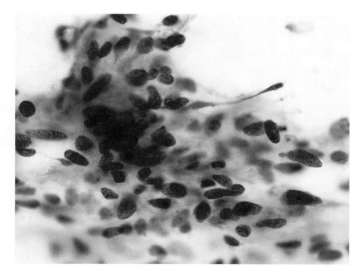

Fig. 2.12 An example of sarcoma: leiomyosarcoma showing cohesive spindle and pleomorphic cells with significant nuclear atypia (Papanicolaou stain)

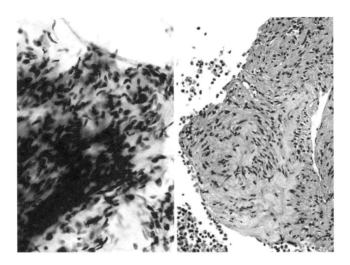

Fig. 2.13 An example of diagnostic traps: schwannoma with ancient change showing nuclear atypia characterized by hyperchromasia and pleomorphism, superficially resembling spindle cell sarcoma. The lack of mitotic figures and the presence of nuclear palisading in the cell block are diagnostic clues (*left*, Papanicolaou stain; *right*, H&E-stained cell block)

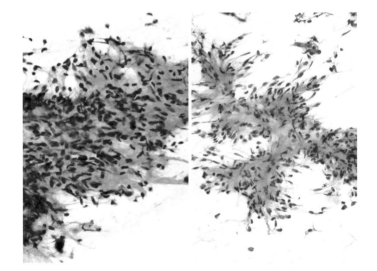

Fig. 2.14 An example of diagnostic traps: nodular fasciitis showing spindle cell proliferation admixed with myxoid stroma, resembling low-grade fibromyxoid sarcoma. Clinical history, superficial location, and feathery or tissue culture-like appearance in smear are diagnostic clues (Papanicolaou stain)

General Strategies of Sample Triage (Fig. 2.1)

- If smears show features suspicious for granuloma or a possible infectious etiology, subsequent aspirates should be collected for the cell block for better architectural assessment and special stains (such as GMS and AFB). In addition, fresh aspirates should be collected sterilely for microorganism cultures.

- If smears of a malignant tumor show cytologic features suggestive of an epithelial or melanocytic lineage, cell block material may be obtained for further workup, especially for lesions in which histologic architectural features are crucial for further evaluation or when immunostaining is anticipated during on-site evaluation.

- If smears show cytologic features suggestive of a mesenchymal tumor, a concurrent core needle biopsy is preferred because core tissue shows architectural relationship between tumor cells and an extracellular component and is ideal for optimal diagnosis of a mesenchymal lesion. In general, mesenchymal lesions have a low aspiration yield compared to epithelial tumors.

- If small round blue cell tumors are found in pediatric patients, collecting material for cytogenetic study is critical. The sample type can be fresh cells in sterile solution, core biopsy, cell block, unstained smear, Diff-Quik-stained smear, or cytospins.

- If smears from a patient with a clinical suspicion of primary lymphoma show cytologic features of lymphoid nature, the next step is to determine whether it is non-Hodgkin lymphoma or Hodgkin lymphoma because the strategy of sample triage for the two entities is different. Of note, low-grade B-cell lymphoma may cytologically overlap with reactive lymphocytes; thus, a lesion containing "reactive-appearing" lymphocytes but with a clinical suspicion of lymphoma should also be worked up to rule out lymphoma.

- If a lesion has clinical or cytologic suspicion of non-Hodgkin lymphoma or plasma cell neoplasm or myeloid malignancy, priority should be given to collect sufficient fresh cells in the cell-preservative medium for flow cytometric immunophenotyping. For these neoplasms in a recurrent setting, a cytologic evaluation combined with flow cytometric immunophenotyping and Ki67 immunostaining on a cytospin is usually sufficient to make a diagnosis; a core needle biopsy is usually not necessary. A diagnosis of large cell lymphoma in a recurrent setting may be made solely on the basis of cytologic features, without immunophenotyping. However, in a primary diagnostic setting, a concurrent core needle biopsy is always necessary, regardless of its subtype, for histologic confirmation, subclassification, and grading.

- If smears show features suspicious for Hodgkin lymphoma or anaplastic large cell lymphoma, a core needle biopsy is the preferred sample type in both primary and recurrent settings. Flow cytometric analysis is essentially of no diagnostic utility.

Sample Preparation for Workup of Non-Hodgkin Lymphoma

- Using a portion of FNA material obtained from the first needle pass for smears and Diff-Quik staining
- Evaluating the smears under a microscope to ensure a lymphoid nature and that non-Hodgkin lymphoma is a possible diagnosis
- Collecting cells from subsequent needle passes into a cell-preservative medium (e.g., RPMI-1640) containing 1 % fetal bovine serum
- Quantifying the cells using an automated counter to determine whether there are sufficient cells for further workup. Five million cells from two needle passes are usually required for a standard lymphoma workup. A cell suspension is primarily used for flow cytometric immunophenotyping to detect aberrant B- and T-cell (sometimes NK-cell) populations.
- In aspirates with a high cellular yield, an aliquot of the cell suspension is processed over Ficoll-Hypaque gradient to enrich the mononuclear cells, which are then centrifuged onto glass slides as cytospin preparation. At MD Anderson, cytospin slides are routinely used for Ki67 staining (to help grade B-cell lymphomas). Occasionally, kappa and lambda stains are performed on cytospins to detect clonality of B-cell population in cases where flow cytometric analysis fails or is not available. CD15 and CD30 stains may be performed on cytospins when classical Hodgkin lymphoma is suspected, but core biopsy or cell block tissue is not available. Extra unstained cytospin slides are stored

in a tumor bank at −80 °C for possible immunostaining or fluorescence in situ hybridization (FISH).
- Collecting material for a cell block is not a priority for hematopoietic lesions, especially non-Hodgkin lymphoma because the lymphoid cells in the block are often crushed. However, an effort to obtain sufficient material for cell block should be made if immunostaining or Epstein–Barr virus in situ hybridization is anticipated.
- If aggregates of tissue or clots are found in the cell-preservative medium but cannot be used for flow cytometric immunophenotyping and cytospin, they should be salvaged to create a cell block.

Suggested Readings

1. Caraway NP. Strategies to diagnose lymphoproliferative disorders by fine-needle aspiration by using ancillary studies. Cancer. 2005;105:432–42.
2. Chen YH, Gong Y. Cytopathology in the diagnosis of lymphoma. In: Nayar R, editor. Cytology in oncology. New York: Springer; 2013. p. 211–40.
3. Cibas ES, Ducatman BS. Cytology: diagnostic principles and clinical correlates. 2nd ed. Edinburgh/London/New York/Oxford/Philadelphia/St Luis/Sydney/Toronto: Elsevier; 2003.
4. DeMay RM. Practical principles of cytopathology. Chicago: American Society of Clinical Pathologists; 1999.
5. Gong Y. Ancillary studies on neoplastic cytologic specimens. In: Nayar R, editor. Cytology in oncology. New York: Springer; 2013. p. 13–29.
6. Gong Y, Caraway N, Gu J, Zaidi T, Fernandez R, Sun X, Huh YO, Katz RL. Evaluation of interphase fluorescence in situ hybridization for the t(14;18)(q32;q21) translocation in the diagnosis of follicular lymphoma on fine-needle aspirates: a comparison with flow cytometry immunophenotyping. Cancer. 2003;99:385–93.
7. Gong Y, Caraway N, Stewart J, Staerkel G. Metastatic ductal adenocarcinoma of the prostate: cytologic features and clinical findings. Am J Clin Pathol. 2006;126:302–9.
8. Gong Y, Joseph T, Sneige N. Validation of commonly used immunostains on cell-transferred cytologic specimens. Cancer. 2005;105:158–64.
9. Gong Y, Sneige N, Guo M, Hicks ME, Moran CA. Transthoracic fine-needle aspiration vs concurrent core needle biopsy in diagnosis of intrathoracic lesions: a retrospective comparison of diagnostic accuracy. Am J Clin Pathol. 2006;125:438–44.

10. Gong Y, Sun X, Michael CW, Attal S, Williamson BA, Bedrossian CW. Immunocytochemistry of serous effusion specimens: a comparison of ThinPrep vs cell block. Diagn Cytopathol. 2003;28:1–5.
11. Gong Y, Symmans WF, Krishnamurthy S, Patel S, Sneige N. Optimal fixation conditions for immunocytochemical analysis of estrogen receptor in cytologic specimens of breast carcinoma. Cancer. 2004;102:34–40.
12. Payne M, Staerkel G, Gong Y. Indeterminate diagnosis in fine-needle aspiration of the pancreas: reasons and clinical implications. Diagn Cytopathol. 2009;37:21–9.
13. Piao Y, Guo M, Gong Y. Diagnostic challenges of metastatic spindle cell melanoma on fine-needle aspiration specimens. Cancer. 2008;114:94–101.
14. Ren R, Guo M, Sneige N, Moran CA, Gong Y. Fine-needle aspiration of adrenal cortical carcinoma: cytologic spectrum and diagnostic challenges. Am J Clin Pathol. 2006;126:389–98.

Chapter 3
Morphologic Evaluation

Morphologic evaluation can be approached by recognizing lineage-specific features and formulating a differential diagnosis for tumors in various lineage-nonspecific groups (Fig. 1.1).

Lineage-Specific Pattern

Determining cell lineage in poorly differentiated tumors is often the first diagnostic step. The general cytologic features of the tumors in the four lineages (i.e., "the Big 4") have been outlined in Chap. 2. Identifying the subtype of a tumor in each lineage category is the second step, followed by detecting the primary origin (Fig. 1.9).

This chapter covers the general features of common subtypes of carcinoma, mesothelioma, and germ cell tumors. In the carcinoma category, the commonly encountered subtypes are adenocarcinoma, squamous carcinoma, neuroendocrine carcinoma, as well as renal cell carcinoma, hepatocellular carcinoma, urothelial carcinoma, and rarely, adrenal cortical carcinoma (Fig. 3.1). The general features of each are described below.

Adenocarcinoma

The individual cells of adenocarcinoma generally have delicate, finely vacuolated cytoplasm, open or vesicular chromatin pattern, and conspicuous or prominent nucleoli, in contrast with the dense cytoplasm and coarse chromatin with inconspicuous nucleoli that

© Springer International Publishing Switzerland 2016
Y. Gong, *Metastatic Neoplasms in Fine-Needle
Aspiration Cytology*, DOI 10.1007/978-3-319-23621-6_3

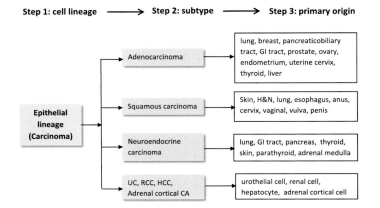

Fig. 3.1 A stepwise approach to cytologic diagnosis of metastatic carcinoma in fine needle aspiration sample: subtyping and primary site determination. Abbreviations: *CA* carcinoma, *GI* gastrointestinal, *HCC* hepatocellular carcinoma, *H&N* head and neck, *RCC* renal cell carcinoma, *UC* urothelial carcinoma

are commonly associated with squamous carcinoma. Although poorly differentiated adenocarcinomas often show disorganized groups and numerous isolated cells with no particular architectural pattern, better differentiated adenocarcinomas tend to show patterns suggesting a primary site. For example, the presence of atypical columnar cells in a necrotic background favors a colorectal origin; high-grade papillary carcinoma in an older woman suggests serous papillary carcinoma of gynecologic origin; and linear arrays or a single-file of plasmacytoid cells is typically seen in lobular breast carcinoma (Fig. 2.8). The five common patterns of adenocarcinoma and the possible primary origins are listed in Fig. 3.2.

Glandular Pattern

Columnar cells with nuclear polarity (i.e., palisading or feathering) and a luminal edge (Fig. 3.3), with a hint of glandular or tubular formation. Smears of glandular structures often form cohesive flat sheets, and the size of the sheet is positively correlated with the size of gland (Fig. 3.4). Note: other types of carcinoma, such as hepatocellular carcinoma, may show glandular-like configurations (Fig. 3.5).

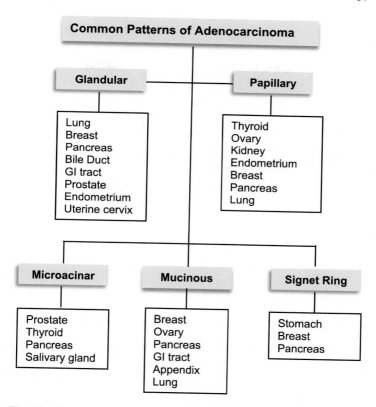

Fig. 3.2 Five common patterns of adenocarcinoma and the common primary origins. Abbreviation: *GI* gastrointestinal

Papillary Pattern

Fingerlike projections with fibrovascular cores and epithelial lining (Figs. 3.6, 3.7, 3.8, and 3.9). Papillary thyroid carcinoma may show a flowerlike configuration (Fig. 3.8) or form flat cohesive sheets on thinner smears (Fig. 3.9). Micropapillary carcinoma usually does not have a true fibrovascular core but shows tight clusters of papillae or small groups (Fig. 3.10). Note: other malignant

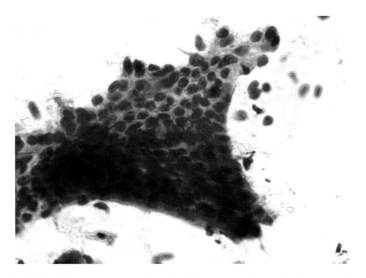

Fig. 3.3 Adenocarcinoma with glandular pattern (example 1): metastatic large duct carcinoma from the prostate showing columnar cells with nuclear palisading and sharp luminal edge (Papanicolaou stain)

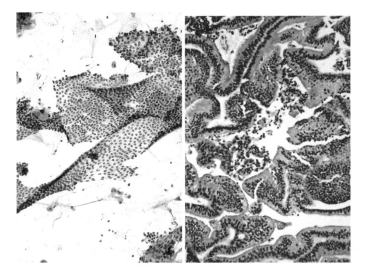

Fig. 3.4 Adenocarcinoma with glandular pattern (example 2): endometrioid carcinoma showing tumor cells that retain nuclear polarity and form cohesive flat sheets. The larger the gland, the larger the sheet is (*left*, Papanicolaou stain; *right*, H&E-stained cell block)

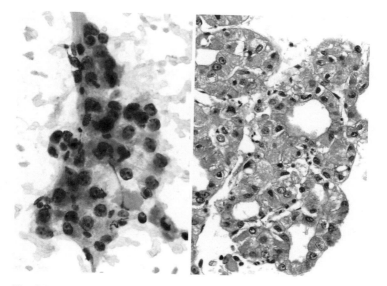

Fig. 3.5 An example of diagnostic traps: hepatocellular carcinoma can form glandular-like cell groups, superficially resembling adenocarcinoma (*left*, Papanicolaou stain; *right*, H&E-stained cell block)

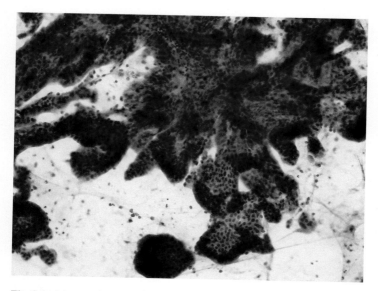

Fig. 3.6 Adenocarcinoma with papillary pattern (example 1): metastatic adenocarcinoma from the pancreas with broad papillary fronds (Papanicolaou stain)

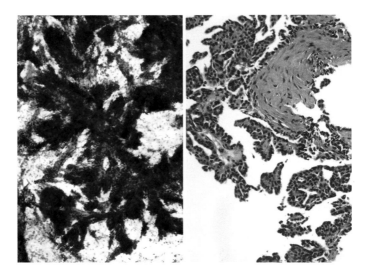

Fig. 3.7 Adenocarcinoma with papillary pattern (example 2): metastatic serious papillary carcinoma from the ovary with delicate papillary fronds and fibrovascular cores (*left*, Papanicolaou stain; *right*, H&E-stained cell block)

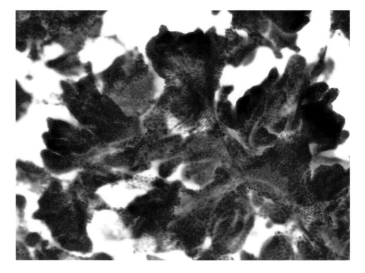

Fig. 3.8 Adenocarcinoma with papillary pattern (example 3): metastatic papillary thyroid carcinoma with large flowerlike papillary fronds and fibrovascular cores (Papanicolaou stain)

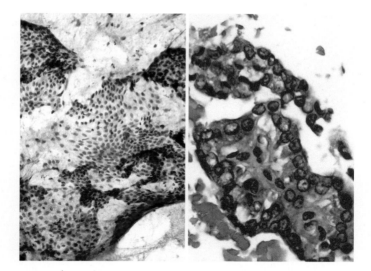

Fig. 3.9 Papillary thyroid carcinomas in thinner area of smear often show flat cohesive sheets. Cell block demonstrates diagnostic nuclear features (*left*, Papanicolaou stain; *right*, H&E-stained cell block)

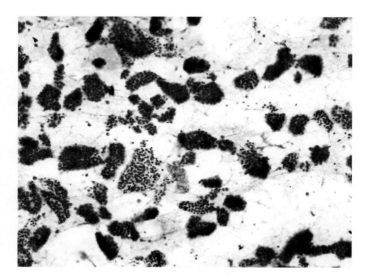

Fig. 3.10 Micropapillary carcinoma usually demonstrates tight clusters of papillae without fibrovascular core. This is a metastatic micropapillary carcinoma from the breast (Papanicolaou stain)

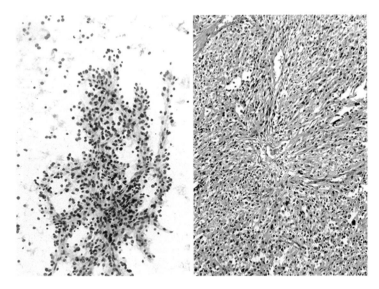

Fig. 3.11 An example of diagnostic traps: a capillary-rich non-papillary tumor (paraganglioma) may yield papillary-like tissue fragments on smear, which can be mistaken for papillary tumor (*left*, Papanicolaou stain; *right*, H&E-stained cell block)

tumors can show true papillary features, such as mesothelioma. Some non-papillary tumors may yield papillary-like tissue fragments on smears if the tumor contains abundant delicate vascular networks, such as paraganglioma (Fig. 3.11).

Microacinar Pattern

Small group of cells forming vague acinar or follicles. This pattern is typically seen in prostatic adenocarcinoma, thyroid follicular carcinoma, acinar cell carcinoma of the pancreas (Figs. 3.12, 3.13, and 3.14), and some salivary gland carcinomas. Note: non-adeno-carcinomas, such as hepatocellular carcinoma and neuroendocrine carcinoma, may show a microacinar-like or rosette-like configuration (Figs. 3.15 and 3.16).

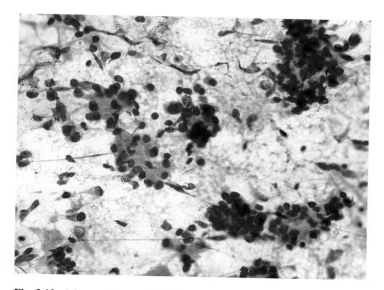

Fig. 3.12 Adenocarcinoma with microacinar pattern (example 1): metastatic prostate carcinoma (Papanicolaou stain)

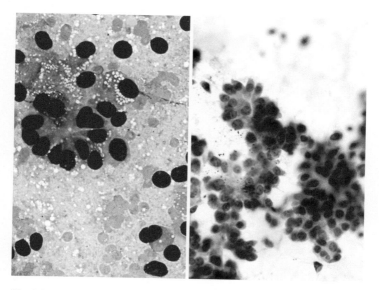

Fig. 3.13 Adenocarcinoma with microacinar pattern (example 2): metastatic pancreatic acinar cell carcinoma (*left*, Diff-Quik stain; *right*, Papanicolaou stain)

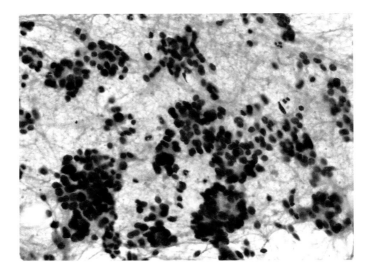

Fig. 3.14 Adenocarcinoma with microacinar pattern (example 3): metastatic follicular thyroid carcinoma (Papanicolaou stain)

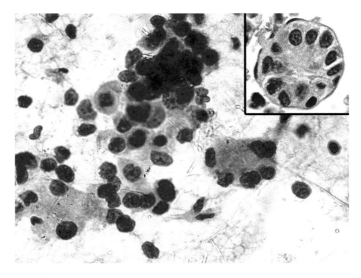

Fig. 3.15 An example of diagnostic traps: non-adenocarcinoma showing microacinar-like configuration as seen in the hepatocellular carcinoma. The hepatoid tumor cells wrapped by endothelial cells are characteristic (Papanicolaou stain; *inset*, H&E-stained cell block)

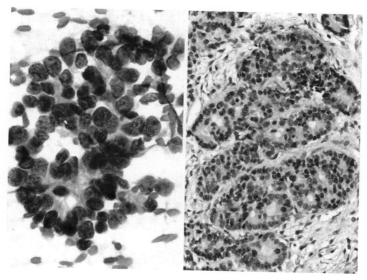

Fig. 3.16 An example of diagnostic traps: non-adenocarcinoma showing microacinar-like configuration as seen in the metastatic neuroendocrine carcinoma (*left*, Papanicolaou stain; *right*, H&E-stained cell block)

Mucinous Pattern

Tumor cells with cytoplasmic mucin, with or without background mucin (Figs. 3.17, 3.18, and 3.19). Note: if a lesion is sampled via endoscopic ultrasound-guided FNA, the background "lesional mucin" should be distinguished from inadvertently sampled mucin from the gastrointestinal tract.

Signet Ring Cell Pattern

Tumor cells with a large cytoplasmic mucin vacuole that compresses the nucleus to one side of the cell (Fig. 3.20). Common primary sites include the stomach, breasts, and pancreas. Note: non-adenocarcinomas, such as vascular tumors and occasionally lymphoma, can show signet ring features (see section "Lineage-Nonspecific Pattern" and Fig. 1.10).

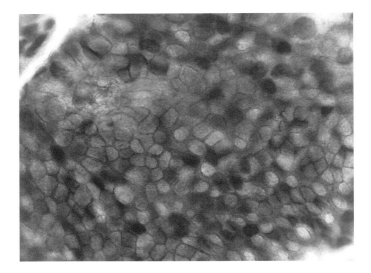

Fig. 3.17 Adenocarcinoma with mucinous pattern (example 1): metastatic adenocarcinoma from the pancreas with evenly distributed intracytoplasmic mucin (Papanicolaou stain)

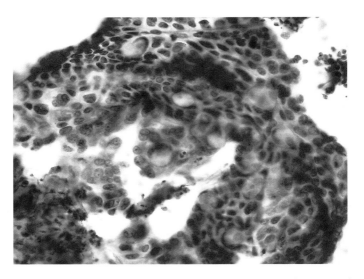

Fig. 3.18 Adenocarcinoma with mucinous pattern (example 2): metastatic adenocarcinoma from the lung with cytoplasmic mucin vacuoles in scattered cells of the cell group (Papanicolaou stain)

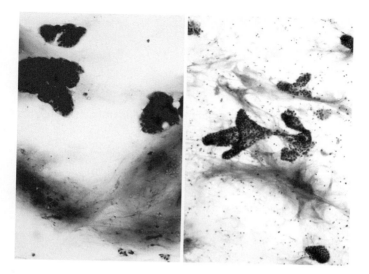

Fig. 3.19 Adenocarcinoma with mucinous pattern (example 3): metastatic mucinous carcinoma from the breast with abundant extracellular mucin in the background (*left*, Diff-Quik stain; *right*, Papanicolaou stain)

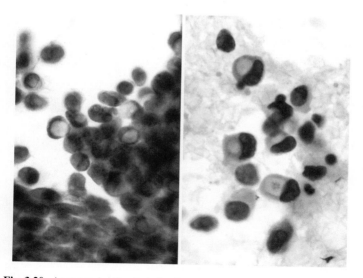

Fig. 3.20 An example of metastatic adenocarcinoma with signet ring cell pattern from breast showing large cytoplasmic mucin vacuole that compresses the nucleus to one side (*left* and *right*, Papanicolaou stain)

Squamous Carcinoma

Well to Moderately Differentiated Squamous Carcinoma (Fig. 3.21):

- Discohesive or single highly pleomorphic or bizarre-appearing ("tadpole") cells
- Keratinized cells: dyskeratotic cells with distinct cell borders, orangeophilic dense cytoplasm (seen in Papanicolaou stain), keratin pearls, and a low N/C ratio in some cells
- Hyperchromatic or pyknotic chromatin and inconspicuous nucleoli
- Anucleate cells and necrotic debris
- Differential diagnosis: epidermal inclusion cyst and benign lesions with squamous metaplasia

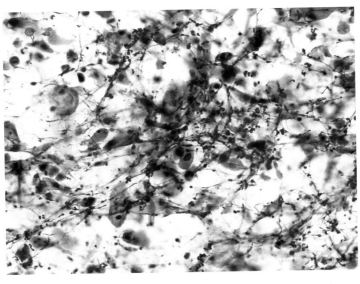

Fig. 3.21 An example of moderately differentiated squamous carcinoma showing bizarre keratinized cells with dense orangeophilic cytoplasm and pyknotic nuclei admixed with anucleate cells and necrotic debris (Papanicolaou stain)

Poorly Differentiated Squamous Carcinoma (Fig. 3.22):

- Large syncytial clusters without keratinized cells and less distinct cell borders compared to better differentiated squamous carcinoma; some tumor cells may have a basaloid appearance
- Relatively uniform cells, higher N/C ratio, and less dense cytoplasm
- Smudging or coarse chromatin with inconspicuous or conspicuous nucleoli
- Necrotic background
- Differential diagnosis: small cell carcinoma, basal cell adenocarcinoma, and basaloid carcinoma of the anal region

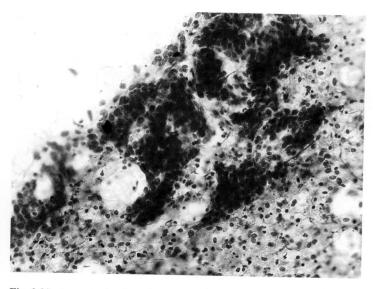

Fig. 3.22 An example of poorly differentiated squamous carcinoma showing syncytial groups of carcinoma cells with smudging chromatin and inconspicuous nucleoli admixed with necrotic debris. There are no keratinized cells (Papanicolaou stain)

Neuroendocrine Carcinoma

(See Chap. 4 for Immunophenotype and Differential Diagnosis of Neuroendocrine Tumors)

Low Grade (Carcinoid and Islet Cell Tumor) (Figs. 3.23 and 3.24):

- Acinar, rosette-like, or trabecular arrangement, numerous loosely cohesive groups and isolated cells
- Uniform round to plasmacytoid cells with eccentrically located nuclei; occasionally spindle cell type
- Occasionally, tiny red cytoplasmic neurosecretory granules (better seen in Diff-Quik stain) and cytoplasmic vacuolization

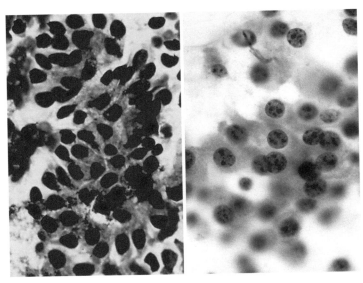

Fig. 3.23 An example of low-grade neuroendocrine carcinoma: metastatic islet cell tumor from pancreas showing uniform, plasmacytoid cells with rosette arrangement. The cells have "salt-and-pepper" chromatin and inconspicuous nucleoli (*left*, Diff-Quik stain; *right*, Papanicolaou stain)

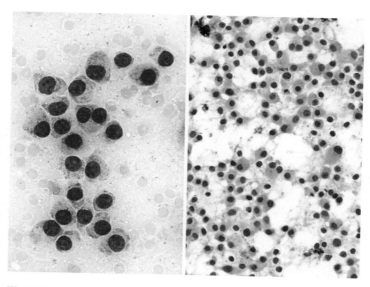

Fig. 3.24 An example of neuroendocrine carcinoma: medullary thyroid carcinoma showing uniform plasmacytoid cells with finely stippled chromatin and indistinct nucleoli. Small neurosecretory granules are seen in *left* panel (*left*, Diff-Quik stain; *right*, Papanicolaou stain)

- Finely stippled chromatin with inconspicuous nucleoli ("salt-and-pepper" appearance) is characteristic. Background amyloid may be seen.
- Increased mitotic figures indicate an higher grade (such as atypical carcinoid).
- Differential diagnosis: tumors with plasmacytoid features (Table 2.3).

High Grade (Small Cell Carcinoma and Merkel Cell Carcinoma) (Fig. 3.25):

- Small- or intermediate-sized round-to-oval cells
- Scant cytoplasm, high N/C ratio, and nuclear molding
- Evenly dispersed chromatin and inconspicuous nucleoli
- Frequent mitotic figures, apoptotic bodies, and crush artifacts (e.g., nuclear streaking)

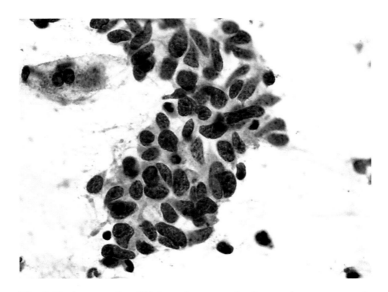

Fig. 3.25 An example of high-grade neuroendocrine carcinoma: metastatic small cell carcinoma from the lung showing small-to-intermediate oval cells with scant cytoplasm and nuclear molding, hyperchromatic but evenly distributed chromatin, and indistinct nucleoli (Papanicolaou stain)

- Background necrosis
- Differential diagnosis: poorly differentiated carcinoma and other small blue cell tumors (see section "Lineage-Nonspecific Pattern," Fig. 1.10)

Urothelial Carcinoma, Renal Cell Carcinoma, Hepatocellular Carcinoma, and Adrenal Cortical Carcinoma

Urothelial Carcinoma (Fig. 3.26):

- Loosely cohesive cell groups or isolated cells
- Epithelioid cells with plasmacytoid or polygonal appearance and scattered "cercariform" cells with a long slender cytoplasmic process and a blunt end

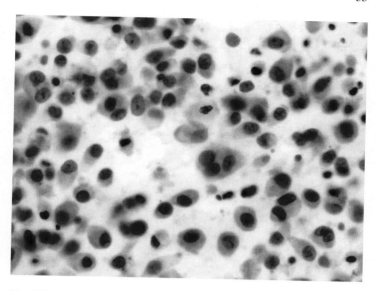

Fig. 3.26 An example of urothelial carcinoma showing loosely cohesive and isolated tumor cells with plasmacytoid features, occasional "cercariform" cells that have fishtail-like end (Papanicolaou stain)

- Occasionally sarcomatoid features
- Differential diagnosis: squamous carcinoma and tumors with plasmacytoid features (Table 2.3)

Renal Cell Carcinoma (see Chap. 4 for Immunophenotype and Differential Diagnosis of Kidney Tumors)

Cytologic features of renal cell carcinomas vary significantly depending on subtype. The most common subtypes are clear cell type and papillary type. Their common features include (Fig. 3.27):

- Tight cell clusters intertwined with capillaries (in clear cell type) or papillary groups (in papillary type), with scattered isolated tumor cells
- Polygonal cells with a moderate to abundant amount of cytoplasm, with a multivacuolated or granular appearance
- Low N/C ratio with abundant cytoplasm

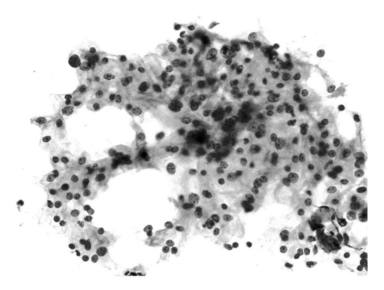

Fig. 3.27 An example of clear cell renal cell carcinoma showing tumor cells with clear cytoplasm that often intertwine with capillaries in tight tissue fragments (Papanicolaou stain)

- Cytoplasmic hyaline globules may be seen
- Depending on tumor grade, the nucleus ranges from bland or small round to bizarre or large pleomorphic and the nucleolus ranges from inconspicuous to prominent
- Differential diagnosis: for clear cell renal cell carcinoma, renal parenchyma (glomeruli and proximal renal tubular cells), benign renal tumors (oncocytoma and angiomyolipoma), chromophobe renal cell carcinoma, adrenal cortical tumors, benign hepatocytes, and hepatocytic tumors; for papillary renal cell carcinoma, other papillary tumors

Chromophobe renal cell carcinoma is less commonly encountered and typically shows hyperchromatic chromatin and perinuclear pale zones. The differential diagnosis includes clear cell renal cell carcinoma and renal oncocytoma.

Collecting duct carcinoma and medullary carcinoma are rare and show high-grade cytologic features. Sarcomatoid component with high-grade spindle and pleomorphic cells can be seen in various proportions in a renal cell carcinoma. The differential diagnosis includes urothelial carcinoma in the renal pelvis and metastatic high-grade tumors.

Hepatocellular Carcinoma (Figs. 3.15 and 3.28):

- Cohesively and discohesively arranged hepatoid atypical cells.
- Thick cords, nests, and acinar groups wrapped by endothelial cells or capillaries traversing tissue fragments are characteristic.
- Individual hepatoid cells are polygonal with moderate to abundant granular cytoplasm, occasionally cytoplasmic bile pigments, and hyaline globules.

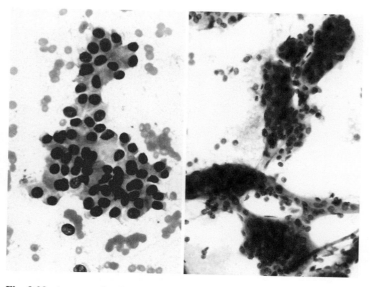

Fig. 3.28 An example of well-differentiated hepatocellular carcinoma showing atypical hepatoid cells with moderate amount of granular cytoplasm. The cells form thick cords and nests that are wrapped by endothelial cells (*left*, Diff-Quik stain; *right*, Papanicolaou stain)

- Increased N/C ratio and may appear monomorphic
- Round central nuclei with inconspicuous to prominent nucleoli
- Isolated cells and significant pleomorphism are usually associated with poorly differentiated tumors
- Differential diagnosis: reactive change of hepatocytes, hepatic adenoma, focal nodular hyperplasia, renal cell carcinoma, adrenal cortical tumors, and metastatic carcinomas

Adrenal Cortical Carcinoma (Fig. 3.29):

- Hypercellular with numerous isolated cells or loosely cohesive clusters
- Round to polygonal cells (occasional sarcomatoid appearance) with intact cell borders and an abundant cytoplasm that can be bubbly, multivacuolated, or granular

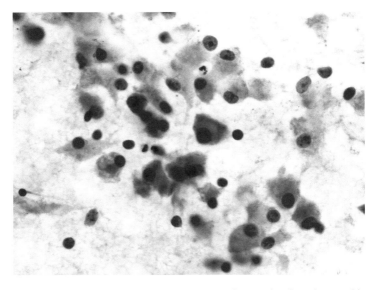

Fig. 3.29 An example of adrenal cortical carcinoma showing pleomorphic malignant cells with abundant granular cytoplasm, arranged in loosely cohesive or single cell fashion (Papanicolaou stain)

- Various degrees of nuclear atypia, pleomorphism, mitosis, and necrosis depending on tumor grade
- Differential diagnosis: adrenal cortical adenoma, pheochromocytoma, renal cell carcinoma, hepatocytic tumors, and metastatic tumors

Mesothelioma (Fig. 3.30)

- Flat cell sheets, isolated cells, and some tight cell clusters
- Large polygonal cells with ruffled edges and prominent intercellular spaces ("windows")
- Occasional spindle cell type (sarcomatoid) or biphasic
- Cytoplasm is dense (especially in the perinuclear area); increased N/C ratio
- Round centrally located nuclei with prominent nucleoli

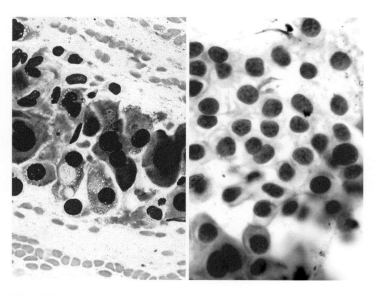

Fig. 3.30 An example of mesothelioma showing large polygonal cells with ruffle edge and prominent intercellular spaces ("windows") (*left*, Diff-Quik stain; *right*, Papanicolaou stain)

- Differential diagnosis: adenocarcinoma and other epithelioid tumors (see section "Lineage-Nonspecific Pattern" in Chap. 3 and Fig. 1.10)

Germating *Germ Cell Tumors*

(See Chap. 4 for Immunophenotype and Differential Diagnosis of Germ Cell Tumors)

Germ cell tumors include seminoma/dysgerminoma, embryonal carcinoma, yolk sac tumor, teratomas, and choriocarcinoma. A mixture of these tumor types is not uncommon. In cytology practice, seminoma/dysgerminoma is encountered more commonly than other subtypes; its cytologic features are listed below (Fig. 3.31):

- Hypercellular with a discohesive or single cell pattern
- Uniform large round tumor cells admixed with lymphocytes and occasional plasma cells

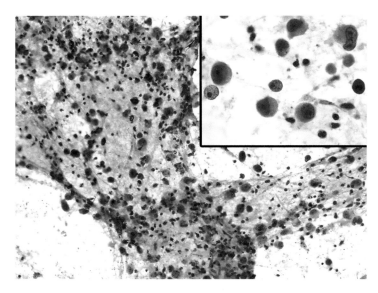

Fig. 3.31 An example of germ cell tumors: seminoma showing discohesive, large round-to-oval malignant cells with pale chromatin and prominent nucleoli and a background of lymphocytes. Occasional naked nuclei are seen (Papanicolaou stain)

- Large round nuclei with pale chromatin, prominent single or multiple nucleoli, and occasional naked nuclei
- Delicate ill-defined cytoplasm and numerous small glycogen vacuoles (seen in Diff-Quik stain)
- "Tigroid" background: stripes due to smearing artifact of glycogen-rich cells (seen in Diff-Quik stain)
- Differential diagnosis: large cell lymphoma, poorly differentiated carcinoma

Lineage-Nonspecific Pattern

The presence of a lineage-nonspecific pattern is a source of diagnostic pitfalls because these groups of malignant tumors show similar cytologic features, although they have various lineages and different histogeneses (Fig. 1.10). A list of differential diagnoses, in conjunction with ancillary studies, is critical for reaching an accurate cytologic diagnosis. The seven most common lineage-nonspecific patterns are listed below.

Tumors with Epithelioid Cell Appearance

- Carcinoma (Fig. 2.2)
- Melanoma (Fig. 2.3)
- Mesothelioma (Fig. 3.30)
- Epithelioid angiosarcoma (Fig. 3.32)
- Epithelioid hemangioendothelioma (Fig. 3.33)
- Epithelioid leiomyosarcoma (Fig. 3.34)
- Epithelioid malignant peripheral nerve sheath tumor
- Epithelioid rhabdomyosarcoma (Fig. 3.35)
- Epithelioid sarcoma
- Osteosarcoma (Fig. 3.36)
- Alveolar soft part sarcoma (Fig. 3.37)

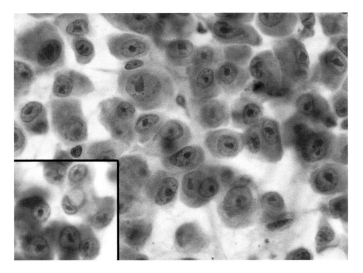

Fig. 3.32 Lineage-nonspecific pattern/epithelioid cell (example 1): epithelioid angiosarcoma showing highly malignant epithelioid cells with occasional intracytoplasmic vacuoles/lumina (*inset*) (Papanicolaou stain)

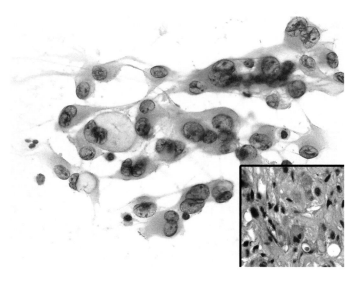

Fig. 3.33 Lineage-nonspecific pattern/epithelioid cell (example 2): epithelioid hemangioendothelioma with cytoplasmic vacuoles/lumina containing red blood cells and myxochondroid matrix (Papanicolaou stain; *inset*, H&E-stained cell block)

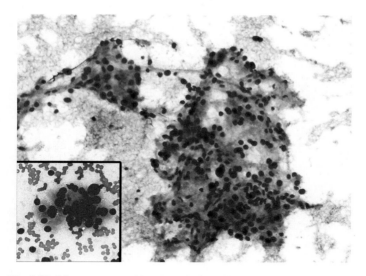

Fig. 3.34 Lineage-nonspecific pattern/epithelioid cell (example 3): epithelioid leiomyosarcoma (Papanicolaou stain; *inset*, Diff-Quik stain)

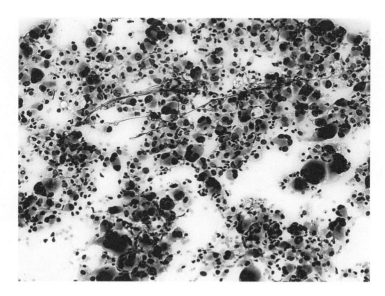

Fig. 3.35 Lineage-nonspecific pattern/epithelioid cell (example 4): epithelioid rhabdomyosarcoma (Diff-Quik stain)

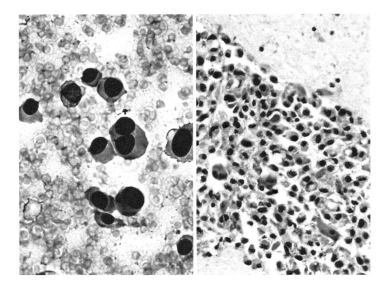

Fig. 3.36 Lineage-nonspecific pattern/epithelioid cell (example 5): osteosarcoma (*left*, Diff-Quik stain; *right*, H&E-stained cell block)

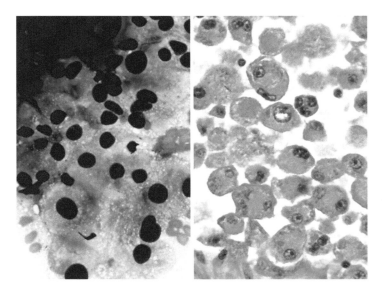

Fig. 3.37 Lineage-nonspecific pattern/epithelioid cell (example 6): alveolar soft part sarcoma showing large, round to polygonal epithelioid cells with prominent nucleoli (*left*, Diff-Quik stain; *right*, H&E-stained cell block)

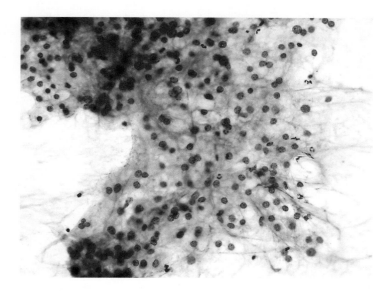

Fig. 3.38 Lineage-nonspecific pattern/epithelioid cell (example 7): chordoma showing epithelioid cells with clear and bubbly cytoplasm, reminiscent of clear cell renal cell carcinoma (Papanicolaou stain)

- Biphasic synovial sarcoma
- Chordoma (Fig. 3.38)
- Epithelioid gastrointestinal stromal tumor (Fig. 3.39)
- Paraganglioma (Fig. 3.40)
- Seminoma (Figs. 3.31 and 3.41)
- Large cell lymphoma (Fig. 2.10)
- Plasma cell neoplasms (Fig. 2.7)

Tumors with Spindle Cell Appearance

(See Chap. 4 for Immunophenotype and Differential Diagnosis of Spindle Cell Malignancies)

- Sarcoma (Figs. 3.42 and 3.43)
- Gastrointestinal stromal tumor (Fig. 3.44)
- Spindle cell carcinoma (Figs. 3.45 and 3.46)

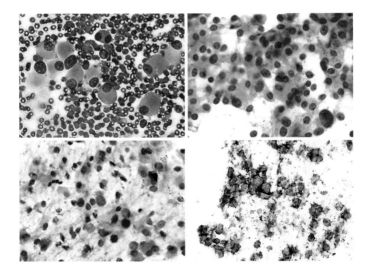

Fig. 3.39 Lineage-nonspecific pattern/epithelioid cell (example 8): epithelioid gastrointestinal stromal tumor, confirmed by positive DOG1 staining (*left upper*, Diff-Quik stain; *right upper*, Papanicolaou stain; *left lower*, H&E stain; *right lower*: DOG1 stain)

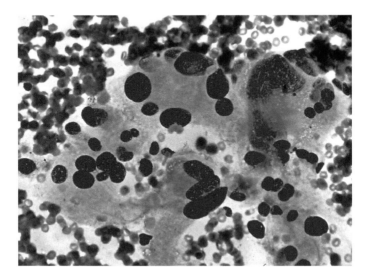

Fig. 3.40 Lineage-nonspecific pattern/epithelioid cell (example 9): paraganglioma showing markedly pleomorphic epithelioid cells forming loosely cohesive acinar-like clusters (Diff-Quik stain)

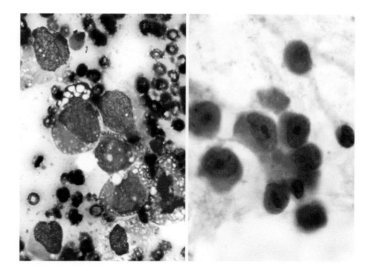

Fig. 3.41 Lineage-nonspecific pattern/epithelioid cell (example 10): seminoma showing large round poorly cohesive epithelioid cells with pale chromatin and prominent nucleoli and numerous small cytoplasmic vacuoles (*left*, Diff-Quik stain; *right*, Papanicolaou stain)

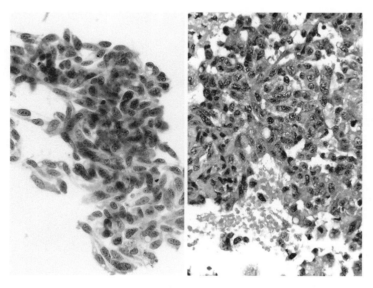

Fig. 3.42 Lineage-nonspecific pattern/spindle cell (example 1): angiosarcoma (*left*, Papanicolaou stain; *right*, H&E-stained cell block)

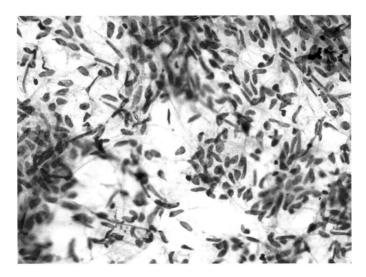

Fig. 3.43 Lineage-nonspecific pattern/spindle cell (example 2): synovial sarcoma, monomorphic (Papanicolaou stain)

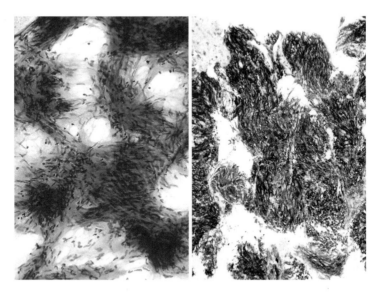

Fig. 3.44 Lineage-nonspecific pattern/spindle cell (example 3): gastrointestinal stromal tumor with positive DOG1 staining on cell block (*left*, Papanicolaou stain; *right*, DOG1 stain)

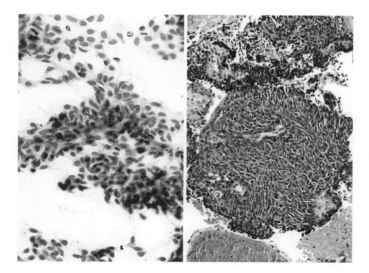

Fig. 3.45 Lineage-nonspecific pattern/spindle cell (example 4): metastatic squamous carcinoma from the lung with spindle cell features (*left*, Papanicolaou stain; *right*, H&E-stained cell block)

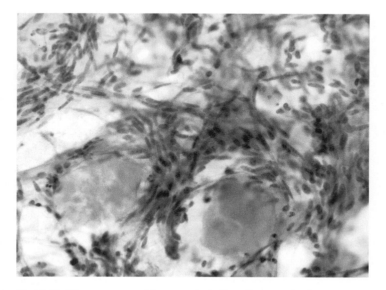

Fig. 3.46 Lineage-nonspecific pattern/spindle cell (example 5): metastatic spindle cell medullary thyroid carcinoma with homogenous amyloid material in the background (Papanicolaou stain)

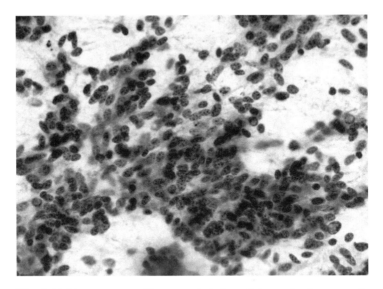

Fig. 3.47 Lineage-nonspecific pattern/spindle cell (example 6): metastatic neuroendocrine carcinoma from the pancreas with spindle cell features and characteristic "salt-and-pepper" chromatin pattern (Papanicolaou stain)

- Neuroendocrine tumors (Figs. 3.47 and 3.48)
- Spindle cell melanoma (Figs. 3.49 and 3.50)
- Sarcomatoid mesothelioma
- Follicular dendritic cell sarcoma (Fig. 3.51)

Tumors with Small Cell Appearance

(See Chap. 4 for Immunophenotype and Differential Diagnosis of Small Round Blue Cell Tumors)

- Small cell carcinoma (Figs. 3.25 and 3.52)
- Merkel cell carcinoma (Fig. 3.53)
- Ewing sarcoma/primitive neuroectodermal tumor (Fig. 3.54)
- Synovial sarcoma
- Rhabdomyosarcoma (Fig. 3.55)

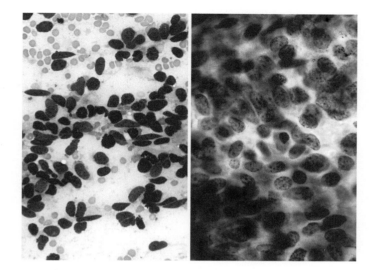

Fig. 3.48 Lineage-nonspecific pattern/spindle cell (example 7): metastatic small cell carcinoma from the lung with spindle cell features (*left*, Diff-Quik stain; *right*, Papanicolaou stain)

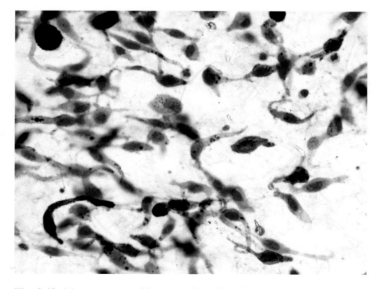

Fig. 3.49 Lineage-nonspecific pattern/spindle cell (example 8): spindle cell melanoma with cytoplasmic melanin pigments (Papanicolaou stain)

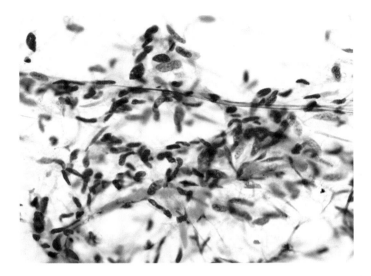

Fig. 3.50 Lineage-nonspecific pattern/spindle cell (example 9): spindle cell melanoma showing bland spindle cells without cytoplasmic melanin pigments, a source of diagnostic pitfalls (Papanicolaou stain)

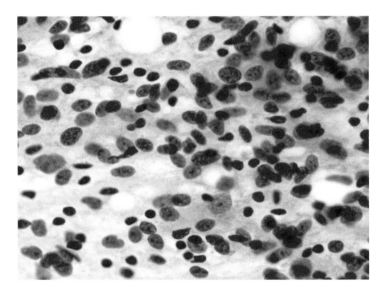

Fig. 3.51 Lineage-nonspecific pattern/spindle cell (example 10): follicular dendritic cell sarcoma showing oval to spindle cells in a background of small lymphocytes (Papanicolaou stain)

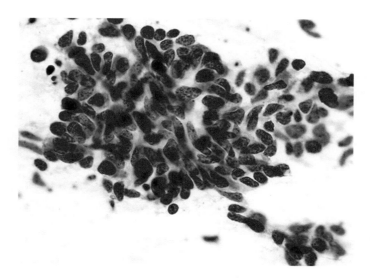

Fig. 3.52 Lineage-nonspecific pattern/small cell (example 1): metastatic small cell carcinoma from the lung showing round-to-oval cells with scant cytoplasm, nuclear molding, and hyperchromatic, evenly distributed chromatin (Papanicolaou stain)

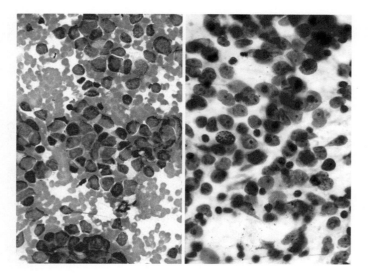

Fig. 3.53 Lineage-nonspecific pattern/small cell (example 2): metastatic Merkel cell carcinoma from the skin showing small- to medium-sized round cells with pale, "powdery" chromatin and micronucleoli, frequent mitotic figures, apoptotic bodies (*left*, Diff-Quik stain; *right*, Papanicolaou stain)

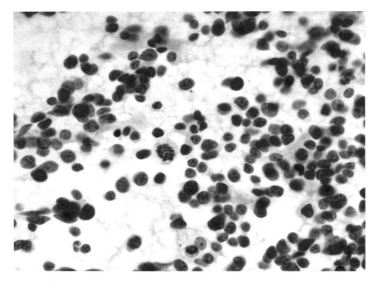

Fig. 3.54 Lineage-nonspecific pattern/small cell (example 3): Ewing sarcoma/primitive neuroectodermal tumor (Papanicolaou stain)

- Small cell osteosarcoma
- Lymphoma (Fig. 2.5)
- Melanoma (Fig. 3.56)
- Neuroblastoma
- Wilms tumor (Fig. 3.57)
- Desmoplastic small round cell tumor (Fig. 3.58)
- Others, including poorly differentiated squamous carcinoma (Fig. 3.59), basaloid squamous carcinoma (Fig. 3.60), solid variant of adenoid cystic carcinoma, basal cell carcinoma (Fig. 3.61), or granulosa cell tumor (Fig. 3.62)

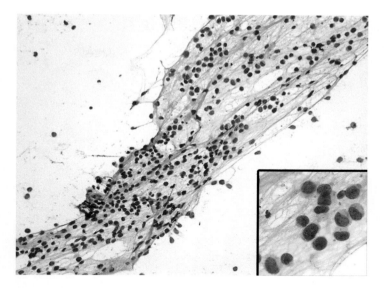

Fig. 3.55 Lineage-nonspecific pattern/small cell (example 4): rhabdomyosarcoma with rhabdoid or plasmacytoid features (Papanicolaou stain)

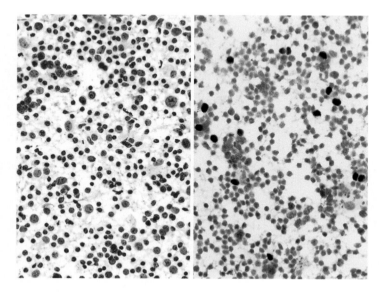

Fig. 3.56 Lineage-nonspecific pattern/small cell (example 5): metastatic melanoma with small cell variant in a lymph node. The small tumor cells closely resemble lymphocytes in the background and the diagnosis was confirmed by positive SOX10 staining on a smear (*left*, Papanicolaou stain; *right*, SOX10 stain)

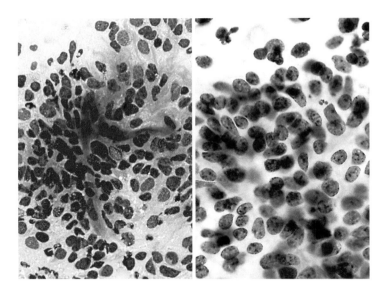

Fig. 3.57 Lineage-nonspecific pattern/small cell (example 6): Wilms' tumor showing uniform small round cells with rosette arrangement (*left*, Diff-Quik stain; *right*, Papanicolaou stain)

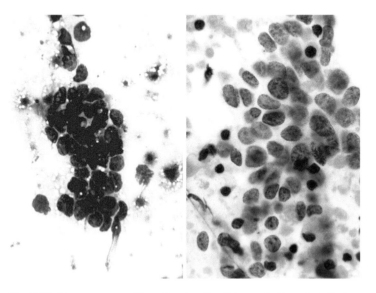

Fig. 3.58 Lineage-nonspecific pattern/small cell (example 7): metastatic desmoplastic small round cell tumor in a neck lymph node (*left*, Diff-Quik stain; *right*, Papanicolaou stain)

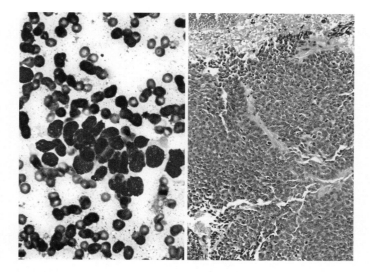

Fig. 3.59 Lineage-nonspecific pattern/small cell (example 8): metastatic poorly differentiated squamous carcinoma in a mediastinal lymph node showing scant cytoplasm and nuclear molding, resembling small cell carcinoma (*left*, Diff-Quik stain; *right*, H&E-stained cell block)

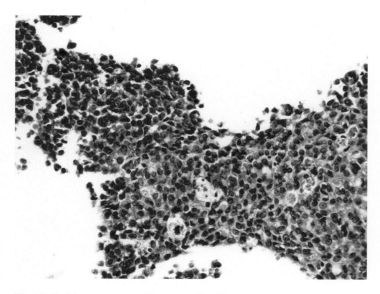

Fig. 3.60 Lineage-nonspecific pattern/small cell (example 9): metastatic basaloid squamous carcinoma from the anus (Papanicolaou stain)

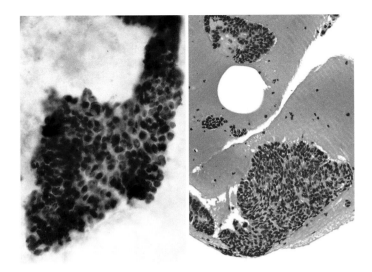

Fig. 3.61 Lineage-nonspecific pattern/small cell (example 10): metastatic basal cell carcinoma from the skin to the lung (*left*, Papanicolaou stain; *right*, H&E-stained cell block)

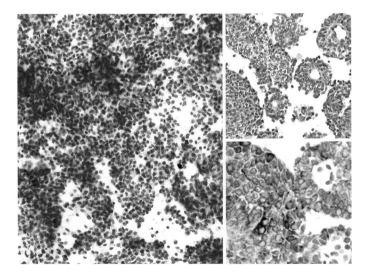

Fig. 3.62 Lineage-nonspecific pattern/small cell (example 11): metastatic adult-type granulosa cell tumor in abdominal soft tissue showing small round cells forming Call–Exner bodies and positive inhibin staining. Nuclear grooves or "coffee bean" nuclei are not readily appreciated (*left*, Papanicolaou stain; *right upper*, H&E-stained cell block; *right lower*, inhibin stain)

Tumors with Pleomorphic Cell Appearance

- Anaplastic carcinoma (Figs. 3.63 and 3.64)
- High-grade sarcoma
- Germ cell tumor, such as choriocarcinoma
- Anaplastic large cell lymphoma (Fig. 3.65)
- Hodgkin lymphoma (Figs. 2.6 and 3.66)
- Melanoma (Fig. 3.67)
- Paraganglioma (Figs. 3.40 and 3.68)

Tumors with Oncocytic Cell Appearance

- Renal cell carcinoma (Fig. 3.69)
- Hepatocellular carcinoma (Fig. 3.70)
- Adrenal cortical carcinoma (Figs. 3.29 and 3.71)

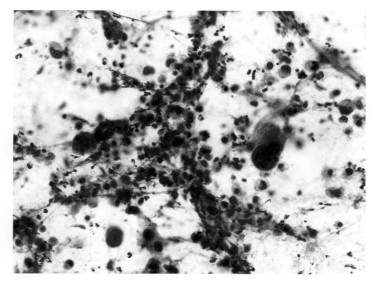

Fig. 3.63 Lineage-nonspecific pattern/pleomorphic cell (example 1): metastatic anaplastic thyroid carcinoma (Papanicolaou stain)

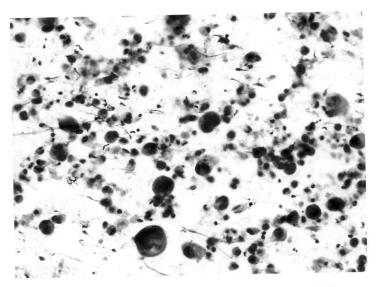

Fig. 3.64 Lineage-nonspecific pattern/pleomorphic cell (example 2): metastatic poorly differentiated esophageal adenocarcinoma (Papanicolaou stain)

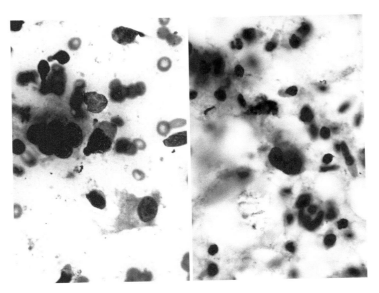

Fig. 3.65 Lineage-nonspecific pattern/pleomorphic cell (example 3): anaplastic large cell lymphoma (*left*, Diff-Quik stain; *right*, Papanicolaou stain)

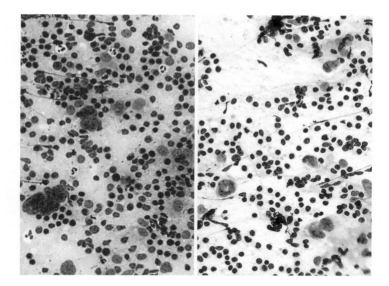

Fig. 3.66 Lineage-nonspecific pattern/pleomorphic cell (example 4): classical Hodgkin lymphoma (*left*, Diff-Quik stain; *right*, Papanicolaou stain)

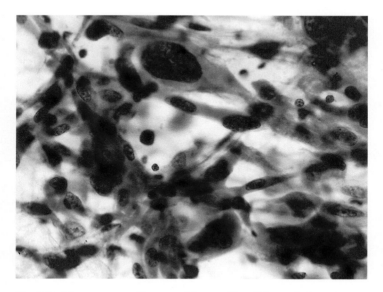

Fig. 3.67 Lineage-nonspecific pattern/pleomorphic cell (example 5): melanoma with anaplastic features (Papanicolaou stain)

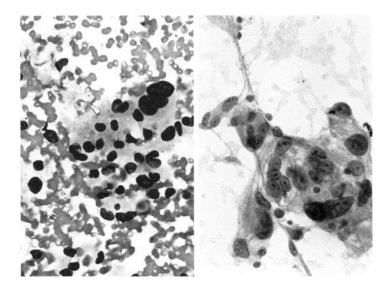

Fig. 3.68 Lineage-nonspecific pattern/pleomorphic cell (example 6): paraganglioma showing markedly pleomorphic epithelioid cells (*left*, Diff-Quik stain; *right*, Papanicolaou stain)

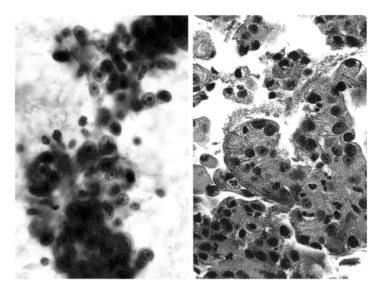

Fig. 3.69 Lineage-nonspecific pattern/oncocytic cell (example 1): metastatic renal cell carcinoma, papillary variant (*left*, Papanicolaou stain; *right*, H&E-stained cell block)

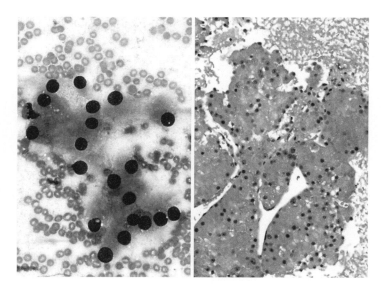

Fig. 3.70 Lineage-nonspecific pattern/ oncocytic cell (example 2): metastatic hepatocellular carcinoma (*left*, Diff-Quik stain; *right*, H&E-stained cell block)

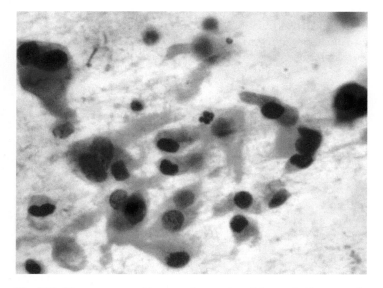

Fig. 3.71 Lineage-nonspecific pattern/oncocytic cell (example 3): metastatic adrenal cortical carcinoma (Papanicolaou stain)

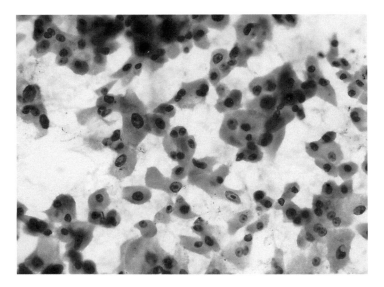

Fig. 3.72 Lineage-nonspecific pattern/ oncocytic cell (example 4): metastatic Hurthle cell carcinoma from the thyroid (Papanicolaou stain)

- Hurthle cell carcinoma of the thyroid (Fig. 3.72)
- Apocrine carcinoma of the breast (Fig. 3.73)
- Acinic cell carcinoma of salivary gland (Fig. 3.74)

Tumors with Clear Cell Appearance

- Renal cell carcinoma (Fig. 3.75)
- Hepatocellular carcinoma (Fig. 3.76)
- Ovarian or endometrial carcinoma (Fig. 3.77)
- Pancreatic endocrine tumor
- Melanoma (Fig. 3.78)
- Seminoma/dysgerminoma (Fig. 3.79)
- Liposarcoma (Fig. 3.80)
- Chondrosarcoma (Fig. 3.81)

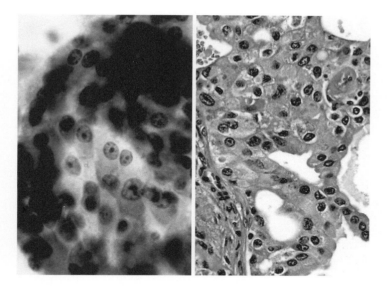

Fig. 3.73 Lineage-nonspecific pattern/oncocytic cell (example 5): metastatic apocrine carcinoma from the breast (*left*, Papanicolaou stain; *right*, H&E-stained cell block)

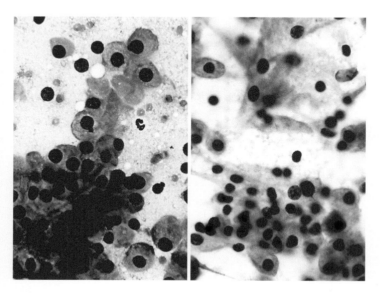

Fig. 3.74 Lineage-nonspecific pattern/ oncocytic cell (example 6): metastatic acinic cell carcinoma of the parotid gland (*left*, Diff-Quik stain; *right*, Papanicolaou stain)

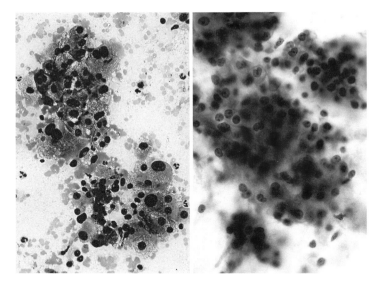

Fig. 3.75 Lineage-nonspecific pattern/clear cell (example 1): metastatic renal cell carcinoma, clear cell type (*left*, Diff-Quik stain; *right*, Papanicolaou stain)

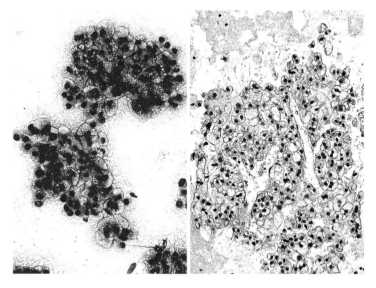

Fig. 3.76 Lineage-nonspecific pattern/clear cell (example 2): hepatocellular carcinoma, clear cell variant (*left*, Diff-Quik stain; *right*, H&E-stained cell block)

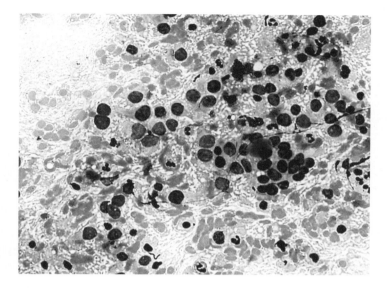

Fig. 3.77 Lineage-nonspecific pattern/clear cell (example 3): metastatic ovarian clear cell carcinoma (Papanicolaou stain)

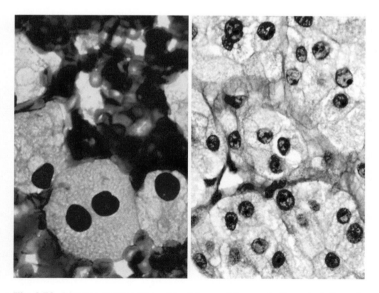

Fig. 3.78 Lineage-nonspecific pattern/clear cell (example 4): metastatic melanoma with clear cell/balloon cell features (*left*, Diff-Quik stain; *right*, H&E-stained cell block)

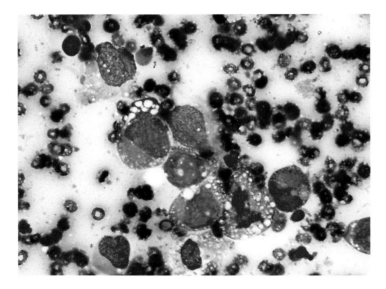

Fig. 3.79 Lineage-nonspecific pattern/clear cell (example 5): metastatic seminoma with numerous clear cytoplasmic vacuoles containing glycogen (Diff-Quik stain)

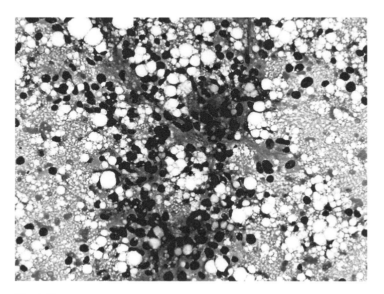

Fig. 3.80 Lineage-nonspecific pattern/clear cell (example 6): metastatic liposarcoma in the liver showing abundant clear cytoplasm containing lipid vacuoles (Diff-Quik stain)

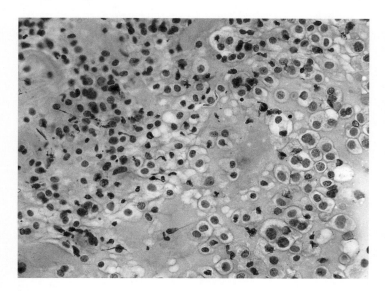

Fig. 3.81 Lineage-nonspecific pattern/clear cell (example 7): chondrosarcoma (Papanicolaou stain)

- Chordoma (Fig. 3.82)
- Squamous carcinoma (Fig. 3.83)
- Carcinoma of the adrenal gland, salivary gland, thyroid, parathyroid, and others (Figs. 3.84, 3.85, and 3.86)

Tumors with Signet Ring Cell Appearance

- Adenocarcinoma (Figs. 3.20 and 3.87)
- Epithelioid angiosarcoma (Figs. 3.32 and 3.88)
- Epithelioid hemangioendothelioma (Fig. 3.89)
- Liposarcoma (lipoblasts) (Fig. 3.90)
- Lymphoma (Figs. 3.91 and 3.92)
- Melanoma (Fig. 3.93)

During morphologic evaluation, caution should be taken to distinguish metastatic malignancies from some benign nonneoplastic

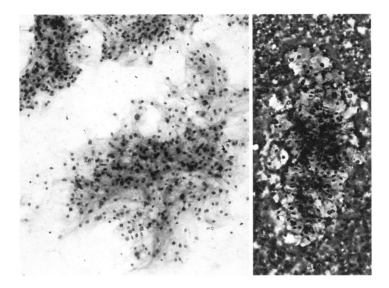

Fig. 3.82 Lineage-nonspecific pattern/clear cell (example 8): chordoma (*left*, Papanicolaou stain; *right*, Diff-Quik stain)

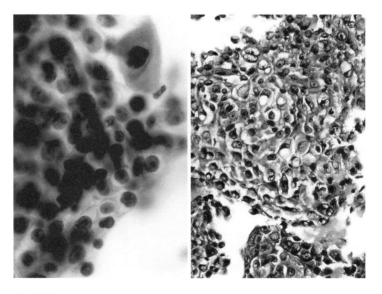

Fig. 3.83 Lineage-nonspecific pattern/clear cell (example 9): squamous carcinoma with clear cell features (*left*, Papanicolaou stain; *right*, H&E-stained cell block)

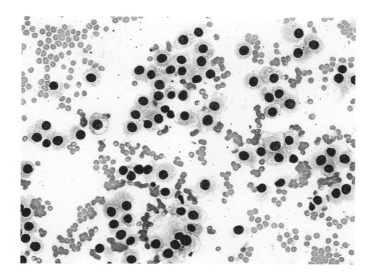

Fig. 3.84 Lineage-nonspecific pattern/clear cell (example 10): metastatic adrenal cortical carcinoma with numerous tiny lipid-rich vacuoles in the cytoplasm (Diff-Quik stain)

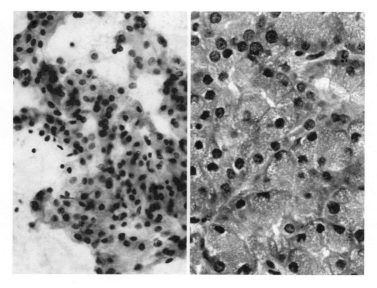

Fig. 3.85 Lineage-nonspecific pattern/clear cell (example 11): metastatic acinic cell carcinoma from parotid gland with clear cell features (*left*, Papanicolaou stain; *right*, H&E-stained cell block)

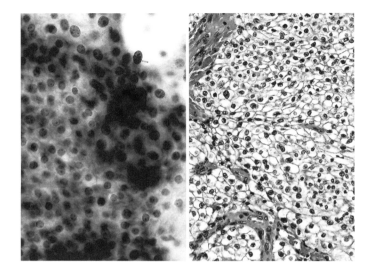

Fig. 3.86 Lineage-nonspecific pattern/clear cell (example 12): parathyroid neoplasm with clear cell features (*left*, Papanicolaou stain; *right*, H&E-stained cell block)

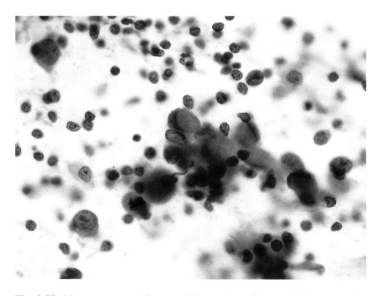

Fig. 3.87 Lineage-nonspecific pattern/signet ring cell (example 1): metastatic signet ring cell adenocarcinoma from the stomach (Papanicolaou stain)

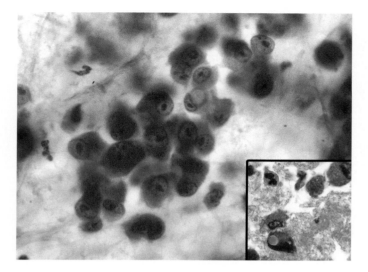

Fig. 3.88 Lineage-nonspecific pattern/signet ring cell (example 2): epithelioid angiosarcoma showing highly atypical epithelioid cells with intracytoplasmic lumina containing red blood cells (Papanicolaou stain; *inset*, H&E-stained cell block)

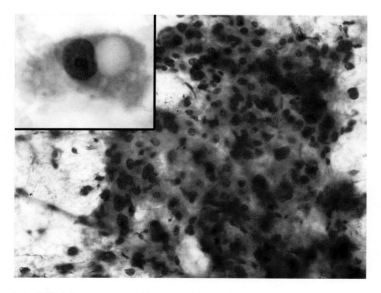

Fig. 3.89 Lineage-nonspecific pattern/signet ring cell (example 3): epithelioid hemangioendothelioma with cytoplasmic lumina and myxochondroid matrix (Papanicolaou stain)

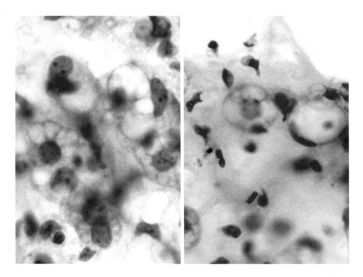

Fig. 3.90 Lineage-nonspecific pattern/signet ring cell (example 4): liposarcoma with signet ring-like tumor cells and lipoblasts that are characterized by several lipid vacuoles indenting or scalloping the nucleus (*left* and *right*, Papanicolaou stain)

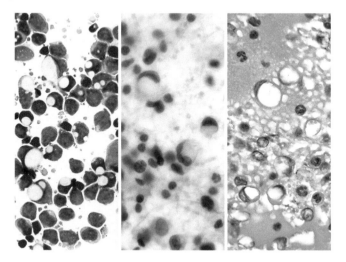

Fig. 3.91 Lineage-nonspecific pattern/signet ring cell (example 5): follicular lymphoma with signet ring cell features. The intracytoplasmic vacuoles may appear clear and empty. The diagnostic clues include that the chromatin pattern of these cells is similar to the adjacent non-vacuolated lymphoid cells and lymphoglandular bodies in the background (*left*, Diff-Quik stain; middle, Papanicolaou stain; *right*, H&E-stained cell block)

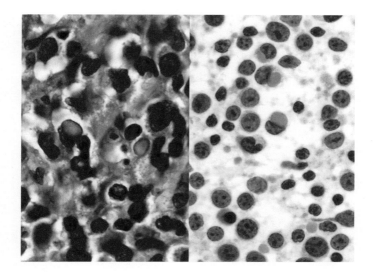

Fig. 3.92 Lineage-nonspecific pattern/signet ring cell (example 6): follicular lymphoma with signet ring cell features containing dense intracytoplasmic hyaline globules. The diagnostic clues include that the chromatin pattern of these cells is similar to the adjacent non-vacuolated lymphoid cells and lymphoglandular bodies in the background (*left*, Diff-Quik stain; *right*, Papanicolaou stain)

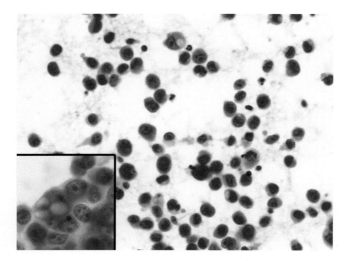

Fig. 3.93 Lineage-nonspecific pattern/signet ring cell (example 7): metastatic melanoma with signet ring cell-like features (Papanicolaou stain)

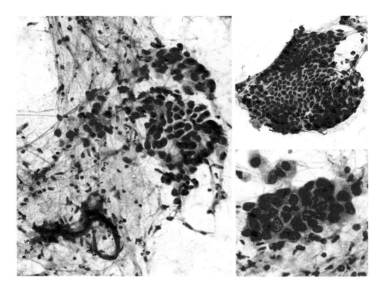

Fig. 3.94 Diagnostic traps (example 1A): an endometriosis in the inguinal region was mistaken for metastatic carcinoma in a lymph node of that region due to the presence of cytologic atypia and lymphohistocytic cells in the background on the smear (Papanicolaou stain)

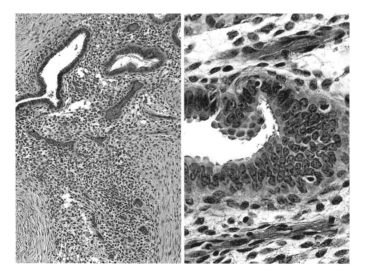

Fig. 3.95 Diagnostic traps (example 1B): the resection specimen of the same lesion shows histologic findings corresponding to cytologic features on FNA smears but consistent with endometriosis of the inguinal soft tissue (H&E-stained resection sample)

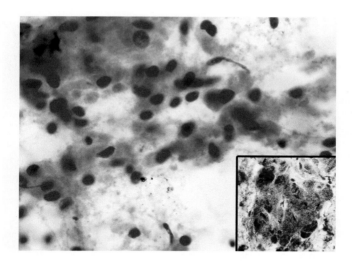

Fig. 3.96 Diagnostic traps (example 2): a granular cell tumor involving the thyroid gland raised a concern for Hurthle cell neoplasm of the thyroid. However, cytoplasmic granules of granular cell tumor are coarser and cell border is less distinct compared to Hurthle cell neoplasm. The diagnosis was confirmed by positive S100 staining on cell block (Papanicolaou stain; *inset*, S100 stain)

lesions or benign tumors, especially when these lesions display some degree of cytologic atypia and similar morphologic patterns. For example, endometriosis with reactive atypia is a common pitfall and can be mistaken for adenocarcinoma (Figs. 3.94 and 3.95). Granular cell tumor can mimic other tumors with oncocytic features (Fig. 3.96). Rarely, thyroid follicular adenoma with dense colloid may resemble adenoid cystic carcinoma (Fig. 3.97).

Melanoma is mostly derived from skin, and its soft tissue counterpart is known as clear cell sarcoma; both show similar cytologic features. Hematopoietic malignancies and mesenchymal malignancies each include a variety of subtypes and morphologic features. Their diagnosis often requires ancillary studies that include not only immunostaining but also flow cytometry, cytogenetic, and sometimes molecular studies (see Chaps. 4–7).

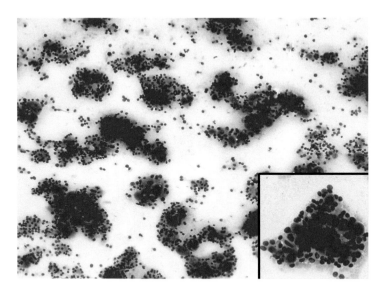

Fig. 3.97 Diagnostic traps (example 3): thyroid follicular neoplasm showing large blobs of dense colloid surrounded by follicular cells, mimicking basement membrane-like hyaline globules surrounded by basaloid cells seen in adenoid cystic carcinoma (Diff-Quik stain)

Suggested Readings

1. Cibas ES, Ducatman BS. Cytology: diagnostic principles and clinical correlates. 2nd ed. Edinburgh/London/New York/Oxford/Philadelphia/St Luis/Sydney/Toronto: Elsevier; 2003.
2. DeMay RM. Practical principles of cytopathology. Chicago: American Society of Clinical Pathologists; 1999.
3. Elsheikh TM, Herzberg AJ, Silverman JF. Fine-needle aspiration cytology of metastatic malignancies involving unusual sites. Am J Clin Pathol. 1997;108:S12–21.
4. Elsheikh TM, Silverman JF. Fine needle aspiration cytology of metastasis to common and unusual sites. Pathol Case Rev. 2001;6:161–72.

5. Gong Y, Caraway N, Stewart J, Staerkel G. Metastatic ductal adenocarcinoma of the prostate: cytologic features and clinical findings. Am J Clin Pathol. 2006;126:302–9.

6. Gong Y, Chao J, Bauer B, Sun X, Chou PM. Primary cutaneous alveolar rhabdomyosarcoma of the perineum. Arch Pathol Lab Med. 2002;126:982–4.

7. Gong Y, DeFrias DV, Nayar R. Pitfalls in fine needle aspiration cytology of extraadrenal paraganglioma. A report of 2 cases. Acta Cytol. 2003;47:1082–6.

8. Gong Y, Krishnamurthy S. Fine-needle aspiration of an unusual case of poorly differentiated insular carcinoma of the thyroid. Diagn Cytopathol. 2005;32:103–7.

9. Gong Y, Sun X, Haines 3rd GK, Pins MR. Renal cell carcinoma, chromophobe type, with collecting duct carcinoma and sarcomatoid components. Arch Pathol Lab Med. 2003;127:e38–40.

10. Ren R, Guo M, Sneige N, Moran CA, Gong Y. Fine-needle aspiration of adrenal cortical carcinoma: cytologic spectrum and diagnostic challenges. Am J Clin Pathol. 2006;126:389–98.

11. Ren R, Sun X, Staerkel G, Sneige N, Gong Y. Fine-needle aspiration cytology of a liver metastasis of follicular dendritic cell sarcoma. Diagn Cytopathol. 2005;32:38–43.

12. Wang J, Katz RL, Stewart J, Landon G, Guo M, Gong Y. Fine-needle aspiration diagnosis of lymphomas with signet ring cell features: potential pitfalls and solutions. Cancer Cytopathol. 2013;121:525–32.

Chapter 4
Immunoperoxidase Studies

As mentioned in the previous chapters, a proper FNA diagnosis often relies on ancillary studies. Immunoperoxidase staining is the most important component in a cytology diagnosis (Fig. 1.1). Like other ancillary studies, immunostaining techniques and markers are continuously developing, and the applications of immunostaining have increased in parallel with the discovery of novel markers in surgical pathology. However, with experience, markers that were initially reported to be specific for a given neoplasm have been found to be less specific than expected. Therefore, it is important to emphasize that no single marker is 100 % sensitive nor 100 % specific for a given tumor and immunostaining should be considered only in the context of a proper differential diagnosis. A small but effective panel should be selected on the basis of the patient's medical history, the clinical and radiologic presentation, and the cytologic features of the lesion.

In addition, prognostic and predictive markers are often requested by clinicians to be tested on FNA samples of metastatic tumors to assess patients' eligibility for certain targeted therapies. Of these, estrogen receptor (ER), progesterone receptor (PR), and human epidermal growth factor receptor 2 (HER2) are the most common markers tested in metastases from patients with a known breast cancer.

Owing to the intrinsic limitations of FNA material, such as sample error, the limited material available for staining, and the lack of intact histologic architecture, immunostaining should be performed and interpreted with caution, using a stepwise approach.

© Springer International Publishing Switzerland 2016   99
Y. Gong, *Metastatic Neoplasms in Fine-Needle
Aspiration Cytology*, DOI 10.1007/978-3-319-23621-6_4

This chapter covers the sample type used for immunostaining in FNA practice, the marker characteristics, the selection and interpretation strategy, and the tiered algorithm. The goal is to judiciously select immunomarkers and use minimal FNA tissue to make an informative diagnosis yet preserve tissue for molecular analysis. Cost-effectiveness is also an important consideration.

Sample Type

- A cell block with decent cellularity, if feasible, is the preferred sample type for immunostaining. This is because the cell block partially retains histologic architecture of a lesion and is processed in a manner similar to that of a surgical pathology specimen. In addition to a needle rinse or separate dedicated pass collected at the time of onsite evaluation, tissue fragments scraped from thick smear are also suitable for making cell block. A pellet obtained from centrifugation is fixed in a mixture of 95 % ethanol and 10 % formalin, embedded in paraffin, and then sectioned. Usually, 8–10 sections are cut upfront, of which the first and the last levels are stained with hematoxylin and eosin (H&E); the unstained sections in between are labeled with a number according to the cutting levels and stored for possible immunostaining or other ancillary studies. The two H&E-stained slides can be used to determine whether tumor cells are present in all the unstained sections and help to ensure that high-priority staining is performed on slides with more tumor cells.
- If a decent cell block is not available, Papanicolaou-stained direct smear may be used if the slides contain a reasonable amount of lesional cells (Figs. 4.1 and 4.2).
- In a situation in which cell block material is not available and the cells of interest are present on only a single Papanicolaou-stained smear, but a panel of markers is needed, a cell-transfer technique can be used to facilitate a multiple marker study using the limited material. In brief, the tissue from a smear is peeled, lifted, and divided into multiple pieces. Each piece is then transferred and firmly adhered to a new slide for a marker

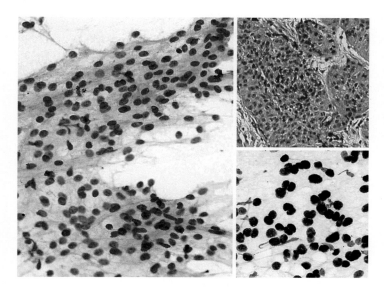

Fig. 4.1 Immunostaining using direct smear when cell block is not available (example 1): smears of a squamous carcinoma do not show typical diagnostic features; the diagnosis was confirmed by positive P63 staining on a smear (*left*, Papanicolaou stain; *right upper*, H&E-stained subsequent resection specimen; *right lower*, P63 stain)

staining. This technique can allow for avoiding a repeat biopsy solely for immunophenotyping of the tumor and thus can reduce patient morbidity and health-care costs.

- In hematopoietic lesions such as lymphoma, cytospin slides containing Ficoll-Hypaque-enriched mononuclear cells may be used for immunostaining (see Chap. 2).
- Technical validation should be performed before routinely using non-cell block preparations for immunostaining to ensure that an expected result can be consistently achieved. For example, at MD Anderson, hormone receptor status is frequently evaluated on direct smears after in-house validation. Papanicolaou-stained direct smears without destaining, but with antigen retrieval, have been proven to be optimal staining conditions (Figs. 4.3 and 4.4).

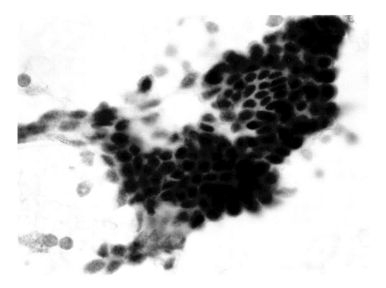

Fig. 4.2 Immunostaining using direct smear when cell block is not available (example 2): positive PAX8 staining on a smear confirms ovarian origin of a metastatic adenocarcinoma in an axillary lymph node, an unusual metastatic pattern (PAX8 stain)

Marker Selection

Although a systematic thought process is important in the cytology diagnosis, immunoperoxidase studies should be tailored on an individual basis and performed judiciously, step by step, to narrow down the differential diagnosis. The goal is to use the smallest necessary panel and yield maximal diagnostic information.

- If a tumor is poorly differentiated, an immunoperoxidase workup may start with lineage determination using a broad spectrum of markers, followed by second and sometimes third panels to define the tumor subtype and primary origin (Fig. 1.1). If a tumor is well to moderately differentiated and shows clear evidence of cell lineage or subtype, then specific markers can be ordered initially. The number of markers depends on the

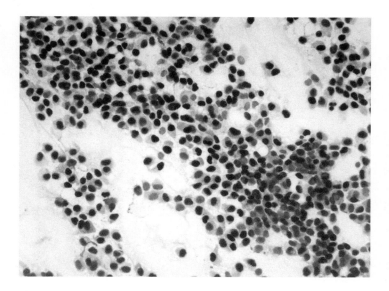

Fig. 4.3 Immunostaining using direct smear when cell block is not available (example 3): positive estrogen receptor staining on a smear of metastatic breast carcinoma; the information was used to guide clinical treatment (estrogen receptor stain)

slides available and priority. Sometimes, a single marker is sufficient for confirmatory purpose if a clinical history of primary tumor is known and the cytologic features are compatible.

- Dual or multiplex staining, in which two or more immunostains are performed on a single slide, can be used in certain cases to save tissue. Dual staining of TTF1 and Napsin A is one of the examples (Fig. 4.5); positive staining seen in either or both markers is often used to confirm a lung primary and an adenocarcinoma subtype.

- The most frequently encountered tumor entities in cytology practice should be considered before selecting markers for detecting rare and unusual tumors.

- Nuclear markers are generally superior to cytoplasmic or membranous markers in cytology preparations. Compared to non-nuclear markers, nuclear staining tends to be more specific and easier to interpret, especially when staining is performed on

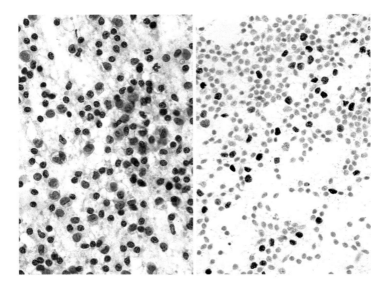

Fig. 4.4 Immunostaining using direct smear when cell block is not available (example 4): positive estrogen receptor staining on a smear of metastatic breast carcinoma in a neck lymph node. The result was used to confirm a diagnosis because the tumor cells are small and bland, reminiscent of the background lymphocytes (*left*, Papanicolaou stain; *right*, estrogen receptor stain)

direct smears in which the intercellular relationship and cell membrane may be distorted or stripped off during smearing (Fig. 4.6). Any true nuclear staining should be considered significant. The commonly used nuclear markers and nonnuclear markers are listed in Tables 4.1 and 4.2, respectively. A few newly discovered yet promising markers are also included. Currently specific markers may become less specific and may be replaced by new markers and new clones that are continually emerging.

• A specific positive result for a particular marker has greater value than a negative result because negative staining may reflect a true negative biologic reaction; however, it may also

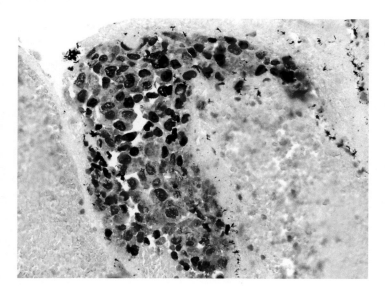

Fig. 4.5 An example of dual or multiplex staining, which allows for multiple markers to be evaluated on the same slides to save tissue: TTF1 (*brown nuclear staining*) and Napsin A (*red cytoplasmic staining*) performed on the same cell block section

result from false negativity. Therefore, marker selection priority should be given to markers that are expected to be positive, although markers that are expected to be negative may be included in a panel.

- If immunophenotypic information about a previous tumor in the same patient is available, selection of positively expressed specific markers to work up the current tumor is helpful to confirm that the two tumors are of the same disease process (Fig. 4.7).
- Marker selection needs knowledge of metastatic pattern. For example, in view of the fact that thyroid gland is an important recipient for metastatic renal cell carcinoma, PAX8 should not be selected to work up a suspected metastatic renal cell carcinoma in the thyroid because tumors originated from both organs express PAX8.

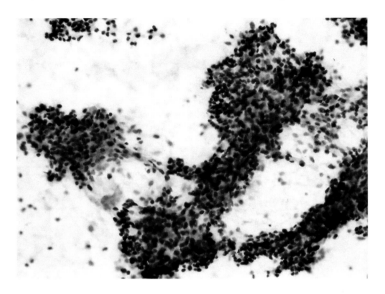

Fig. 4.6 Immunostaining using direct smear when cell block is not available (example 5): positive TTF1 staining on a smear confirms a metastatic papillary thyroid carcinoma in soft tissue of the thigh (TTF1 stain)

Marker Interpretation and Caveats

- Correlation with clinical and radiologic findings and cytologic features.
- Knowledge of the distribution of specific staining in cells (nuclear, cytoplasmic, or membranous).
- Focusing on staining in healthy and viable tumor cells, avoiding degenerated cells or cells in necrotic areas.
- Judicious examination of positive and negative controls that ideally should be processed and stained in the same manner as the test sample at each run of staining.
- Immunostaining on non-cell block preparations, such as direct smears, usually does not have proper control tissue. Extra caution should be taken during interpretation.

Table 4.1 Nuclear markers that are relatively site specific (in alphabetical order)

Nuclear marker	Main application (tumor types/origins)	Selected other tumor types
ALK	Anaplastic large cell lymphoma	Inflammatory myofibroblastic tumor (cytoplasmic staining); lung AdCA with EML4-ALK rearrangement
Brachyury	Chordoma	
Calretinin*	Mesothelioma Adrenal cortical tumors	Sex cord stromal tumors
CDX2	AdCA of the GI tract (lower>upper) AdCA of the pancreaticobiliary tract	Neuroendocrine tumors (GI tract>other sites) Tumors with enteric phenotype (e.g., mucinous AdCA of the ovary, lung, cervix), urinary bladder AdCA, yolk sac tumor
ER	Breast CA	AdCA of gynecologic origin, sweat gland, salivary gland, and lung (rare)
ERG	Vascular tumors	Prostate CA
FLI1	Ewing sarcoma Vascular tumors	Some lymphomas, Merkel cell CA Lung CA, breast CA
GATA3	Urothelial CA Breast CA	Paraganglioma, chromophobe renal cell CA, squamous CA, mesothelioma, pancreaticobiliary AdCA CA of the salivary gland, skin, and pancreas
MDM2, CDK4	Liposarcoma (dedifferentiated types > well differentiated)	Positive for both markers is more specific
MITF	Melanoma of the skin or soft tissue	PEComas, soft tissue tumors with melanocytic differentiation
MyoD1, myogenin	Rhabdomyosarcoma	

(continued)

Table 4.1 (continued)

Nuclear marker	Main application (tumor types/origins)	Selected other tumor types
NKX3.1	Prostate CA	Breast CA (lobular>ductal)
OCT3/4	Seminoma/dysgerminoma and embryonal CA of gonadal or extragonadal sites	
PAX2	Renal cell CA (clear cell, papillary)	AdCA of gynecologic origin (not thyroid or thymic tumors)
PAX5	B-cell lineage lymphomas	Small cell CA (lung>other sites)
PAX8	Renal cell CA (all types)	Urothelial CA (−/+)
	Thyroid CA (papillary/follicular>anaplastic>medullary)	Neuroendocrine tumors of the pancreas, thymic tumors, parathyroid tumors, lymphoma and benign lymphocytes
	Endometrial AdCA, cervical AdCA, ovarian AdCA (nonmucinous>mucinous)	
PR	Breast CA, salivary duct CA	Pancreatic endocrine tumor, solid pseudopapillary tumor
P16*	HPV-associated squamous CA of the cervix, anogenital and oropharyngeal origins (strong and diffuse staining)	Serous CA of gynecologic origin (used analogously to p53 and unrelated to HPV)
P40	Squamous CA	Urothelial CA
P63	Squamous CA	Urothelial CA, thymic tumors, Metaplastic breast carcinoma
Sall4	Germ cell tumors of gonadal or extragonadal sites	
SATB2	AdCA of the lower GI tract	Neuroendocrine tumors of the left colon and rectum, papillary renal cell CA, osteosarcoma
SF1	Adrenal cortical tumors	Sex cord stromal tumors
SOX9	Cartilaginous tumors	

SOX10	Melanoma of the skin or soft tissue	Nerve sheath tumors (benign>malignant), some breast CA, salivary gland CA, carcinoid tumors
SOX11	Mantle cell lymphoma	Lymphoblastic lymphoma, Burkitt lymphoma, Merkel cell CA
S100*	Melanoma of the skin or soft tissue	Subset of CA (breast, salivary gland, sweat gland, thyroid origins), granular cell tumor, Langerhans cell histiocytosis, PEComas
	Nerve sheath tumors	Neurofibroma, dendritic cell tumors, chondrosarcoma, chordoma, lipomatous tumors
STAT6	Solitary fibrous tumor	
TFE3	Alveolar soft part sarcoma	Xp11 translocation renal cell CA, subset of PEComas, epithelioid hemangioendothelioma
TLE1	Synovial sarcoma	Schwannoma, solitary fibrous tumor
TTF1	AdCA of the lung (nonmucinous>mucinous)	Small cell CA (lung>other sites), lung carcinoid, large cell neuroendocrine CA of various sites; positive cytoplasmic TTF1 staining can be seen in hepatocellular CA and benign hepatocytes
	Thyroid CA (papillary, follicular, medullary)	AdCA of gynecologic origin
WT1	Ovarian serous CA, mesothelioma	Primary peritoneal serous CA, Wilms tumor, DPSRCT, endometrial stromal sarcoma

Abbreviations of tumor entities: *AdCA* adenocarcinoma, *CA* carcinoma, *DPSRCT* desmoplastic small round cell tumor, *GI* gastrointestinal, GI*ST* gastrointestinal stromal tumor, *PEComas* perivascular epithelioid cell neoplasms (including angiomyolipoma, clear cell sugar tumors, lymphangioleiomyomatosis), *PNET* primitive neuroectodermal tumor

* S100, calretinin, and P16 each show both nuclear and cytoplasmic staining

1) MDM2 and CDK4 are negative for pleomorphic liposarcoma or myxoid/round cell liposarcoma

2) Most melanoma-associated antigens are also present in other melanosome-containing tumors, such as melanoma of soft parts, melanotic nerve sheath tumors, as well as PEComas

3) Both P40 and P63 are expressed in squamous CA of various origins. P40 has higher specificity than P63

Table 4.2 Nonnuclear (cytoplasmic or membranous) markers (in alphabetical order)

Nonnuclear marker	Main application (tumor types/origins)	Selected other tumor types
AFP	Hepatocellular CA	Germ cell tumors
Arginase	Hepatocellular CA	AdCA of the pancreaticobiliary tract (rare)
Calcitonin	Medullary thyroid CA	
CD30	Classical Hodgkin lymphoma, anaplastic large cell lymphoma	Embryonal CA
CD31, FactorVIII	Vascular tumors	
CD38	Plasma cell neoplasms	Some B-cell lymphomas
CD138	Plasma cell neoplasms	Some carcinomas, sarcomas, lymphomas
CD117 (cKit)	GIST, seminoma/dysgerminoma, myeloid sarcoma	Renal cell CA (chromophobe), plasma cell neoplasms, melanoma, PEComas, renal oncocytoma, thymic CA, adenoid cystic CA of salivary gland
CDH17	AdCA of the GI tract (lower > upper)	Pancreatic AdCA, neuroendocrine tumors of the GI tract and pancreas
Chromogranin	Neuroendocrine tumors	
CK20	AdCA of the colon and rectum, Merkel cell CA of the skin (perinuclear dot pattern)	
CK5/6	Squamous CA, urothelial CA Mesothelioma	Metaplastic breast carcinoma
CK903	Squamous CA, urothelial CA	Metasplastic breast carcinoma
Desmin, MSA	Smooth muscle and skeletal muscle tumors	Desmin also + in mesothelial cells (benign > malignant) and non-myogenic tumors (DPSRCT, blastemal component of Wilms tumor)

D2-40	Mesothelioma, seminoma	Embryonal CA
DOG1	GIST	Acinic cell CA of salivary gland
GCDFP, mammaglobin	Breast CA	Subset of salivary duct and sweat gland and lung CA
Glypican3	Hepatocellular CA	Yolk sac tumor
HepPar1	Hepatocellular CA	CA with hepatoid phenotype in extrahepatic sites, AdCA of the stomach and esophagus
HMB45	Melanoma of the skin or soft tissue	PEComas, melanotic schwannoma
Inhibin	Adrenal cortical tumors	Sex cord stromal tumors, granular cell tumor
Melan A/MART1	Melanoma of the skin or soft tissue	Adrenal cortical tumors and sex cord stromal tumors if using Melan A (clone A103), PEComas
Mesothelin	Mesothelioma	AdCA of various sites
Napsin A	AdCA of the lung	Renal cell CA (papillary>clear cell), ovarian clear cell CA, rare thyroid papillary CA
NY-ESO-1	Myxoid/round cell liposarcoma	Breast cancer
	Synovial sarcoma	
PLAP	Germ cell tumors of gonadal or extragonadal sites	
PSA, PAP	Prostate CA	Breast and salivary gland CA. PSA is more specific but less sensitive than PAP
Prostein (P501S)	Prostate CA	
RCC	Renal cell CA (clear cell, papillary)	Adrenal cortical CA, breast CA

(continued)

Table 4.2 (continued)

Nonnuclear marker	Main application (tumor types/origins)	Selected other tumor types
SMA	Smooth muscle tumors	Myofibroblastic lesions
Synaptophysin	Neuroendocrine tumors	Neuroblastoma, Ewing sarcoma/PNET, DPSRCT, adrenal cortical tumors, solid pseudopapillary tumor of pancreas
Thrombomodulin	Urothelial CA	Mesothelioma
Thyroglobulin	Thyroid CA (papillary, follicular)	
PTH	Parathyroid tumors	
Uroplakin	Urothelial CA	
Villin	AdCA of the GI tract (lower>upper)	Tumors with enteric phenotype (e.g., mucinous AdCA of the ovary, lung), urinary bladder AdCA, endometrial CA, yolk sac tumor

Abbreviations of tumor entities: *AdCA* adenocarcinoma, *CA* carcinoma, *DPSRCT* desmoplastic small round cell tumor, *GI* gastrointestinal, *GIST* gastrointestinal stromal tumor, *PEComas* perivascular epithelioid cell neoplasms (including angiomyolipoma, clear cell sugar tumors, and lymphangioleiomyomatosis), *PNET* primitive neuroectodermal tumor

1) GCDFP and mammaglobin both have low sensitivity for breast carcinoma. GCDFP15 expression is more often in lobular carcinoma than ductal carcinoma of the breast. Occasionally, mammaglobin may be positive in endometrial carcinoma and GCDFP15 may be positive in lung adenocarcinoma

2) Both arginase and HepPar1 are positive for benign liver cells and hepatocellular carcinoma. Arginase is more sensitive and specific than HepPar1 and Glypican3 for hepatocellular carcinoma, especially for poorly differentiated one. Arginase expression is usually negative in hepatoid carcinoma in extrahepatic sites

3) Glypican3 is positive in well-differentiated hepatocellular carcinoma but negative in benign hepatic nodule

4) RCC marker has low sensitivity and specificity for renal cell carcinoma

5) Villin has less sensitivity than CDX2 for gastrointestinal tumors

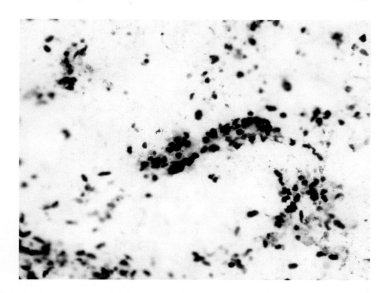

Fig. 4.7 Immunostaining using direct smear when cell block is not available (example 6): positive CDX2 staining on a smear confirms colorectal origin of a metastatic adenocarcinoma in a retroperitoneal lymph node (CDX2 stain)

- Definition of positivity in terms of the percentage of positive lesional cells required may vary for different markers. However, for the interpretation of prognostic and predictive markers such as ER, PR, and HER2, standard guidelines should be followed.
- Net results of the entire immunostaining panel should be used when considering a final diagnosis.
- False-negative results are more common than are false-positive results. Therefore, a positive result is generally more meaningful than a negative result.
- False-negative results are largely due to sample error (i.e., scarcity of lesional cells available for immunostaining from a tumor that intrinsically expresses the markers only focally and heterogeneously) and inappropriate preanalytical and analytical factors (e.g., using non-cell block material for immunostaining without technical validation). Certain stains, such as S100,

cannot be reliably assessed on ethanol-fixed preparations, possibly resulting in false-negative findings.

- False-positive results are usually due to erroneous interpretation. The lack of reliable histologic architecture in the aspirated material can cause entrapped benign cells at the aspiration site to be mistaken for tumor cells. For example, an aspirate of a metastatic carcinoma to the lungs may be admixed with entrapped benign bronchial epithelial cells that express TTF-1, potentially leading to the erroneous conclusion that the tumor is focally TTF-1 positive and thus a lung primary. In addition, nonspecific staining is often seen in crowded cell groups of thick smears or in association with the edge effect. It can cause a false-positive interpretation. Occasionally, staining of the cytoplasm overlying a nucleus which is actually negative for a nuclear marker may appear weak reactivity in the nucleus due to the integrity of the cells and the three-dimensional nature of the cells on the smear.

- Be aware of some caveats that may be associated with TTF1, CDX2, and PAX8, the most commonly used nuclear markers in cytology practice. For example, CDX2 may be positive in adenocarcinomas from the lung, ovary, and urinary bladder with enteric phenotype and yolk sac tumor. Lung adenocarcinomas with enteric phenotype or mucinous subtype usually have lower frequency of TTF1 expression than those with nonmucinous subtype. Likewise, ovarian adenocarcinomas with enteric phenotype or mucinous subtype less likely express PAX8 than those with nonmucinous subtype. In addition, when a distinction between thyroid and parathyroid or between thyroid and thymic tumor is needed, PAX8 should not be selected because lesions from these origins can express PAX8. PAX8 can also be positive in lymphoid cells; thus caution should be taken when using PAX8 to detect metastatic carcinoma in lymph node sample. In addition to carcinoma originated from renal, thyroid, and gynecologic organs, PAX8 is frequently expressed in well-differentiated pancreatic endocrine tumor. Lastly, PAX8 is usually used to distinct renal cell carcinoma (positive) from urothelial carcinoma (negative); however, a subset of upper tract urothelial carcinoma may express PAX8.

Tiered Diagnostic Algorithm of Immunoperoxidase Workup

The tiered approach involves the sequential application of selected markers: the smallest yet most effective panel. The entities listed in the tables of this chapter are the malignant tumors that are most frequently encountered in cytology practice, although a few low-grade and benign lesions are included for the purpose of differential diagnosis. The staining results in the tables are not absolute and may vary depending on variations in the sensitivity and specificity of the antibody used, staining conditions, and tumor differentiation. In general, "−" or "negative" signifies the percentage of positive cases in the 0–10 % range; "−/+" signifies the percentage of positive cases in the 10–50 % range; "+/−" signifies the percentage of positive cases in the 50–70 % range; and "+" or "positive" signifies the percentage of positive cases in the >70 % range.

Determination of Tumor Lineage (Step 1)
(Figs. 1.9 and 4.8)

Even though each diagnostic algorithm differs according to the clinical and cytologic findings, for cases that need to be worked up from lineage determination, the first-tier panel of immunostaining markers includes panCK, melanocytic markers (such as MART1), and a hematopoietic marker (such as CD45) to determine the epithelial, melanocytic, and hematopoietic lineages of the tumor, respectively.

Epithelial Markers

Cytokeratins are present in epithelial cells and are the hallmarks of this lineage. AE1/AE3 used to be considered a first-line screening marker. Although AE1/AE3 is expressed in the majority of epithelial neoplasms, a few exceptions exist. For example, hepatocellular

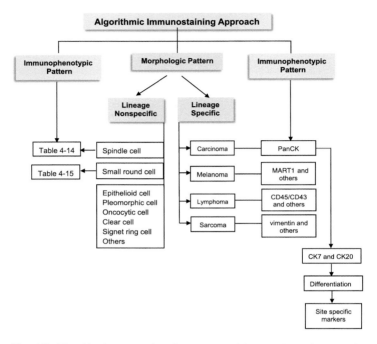

Fig. 4.8 Algorithmic approach to immunoperoxidase workup of metastatic tumors

carcinoma is not recognized by AE1/AE3 because hepatocytes are positive for CK18, which is not included in AE1/AE3 but is included in CAM5.2. Neuroendocrine carcinomas, including small cell carcinoma, variably express both AE1/AE3 and CAM5.2. CAM5.2 is complementary to AE1/AE3 and can recognize the few carcinomas that are missed by AE1/AE3. Therefore, pancytokeratin (panCK), a cocktail of AE1/AE3 and CAM5.2 and other keratins, should be used as a screening cytokeratin in cytology practice.

PanCK greatly increases the screening sensitivity of confirming an epithelial nature of the malignancy; some carcinomas are still negative for this marker (Table 4.3). For renal cell carcinoma, the addition of EMA could be helpful. Adrenal cortical carcinoma frequently lacks expression of panCK or any other epithelial markers, including EMA. Caution should be taken in the interpretation of

Table 4.3 Carcinomas that may show negative panCK staining

Carcinoma type	panCK (%)
Adrenal cortical carcinoma	15 %
Anaplastic thyroid carcinoma	75 %
Embryonal carcinoma	75 %
Hepatocellular carcinoma	80 %
Renal cell carcinoma	80 %
Small cell carcinoma	Variable depending on site
Spindle cell/sarcomatoid carcinoma	Variable depending on site

panCK in small cell carcinoma, in which the degree of panCK expression varies depending on the primary origin and the staining can be focal and subtle because the cells have very little cytoplasm.

On the other hand, non-carcinoma malignancies may show variable expression of panCK, especially tumors with epithelioid appearance, including melanoma, sarcoma, and hematopoietic tumors (Table 4.4). Staining in most of these tumors tends to be focal and weak. However, these could be the traps for the unwary. Of note, mesothelioma and most germ cell tumors (excepting seminoma/dysgerminoma) are epithelial-derived tumors and are positive for panCK.

CK5/6 and CK903 are both high molecular weight keratin, but are not included in panCK. They are reactive to squamous, urothelial, and metaplastic breast carcinomas.

Melanocytic Markers

Commonly used melanocytic markers in cytology practice include MART1, SOX10, MITF, S100, and HMB45. Although S100 is quite sensitive for melanoma in paraffin-embedded tissue sections, it is not very specific and can be expressed in a subset of tumors from different lineages, including carcinomas, sarcomas, and dendritic cell tumors (Table 4.1). In addition, S100 staining on ethanol-fixed preparations may show a false-negative result; thus, it is not a preferred marker in cytology practice. HMB45 has high specificity but relatively low sensitivity. MART1 is often used as a first-line marker. When direct smear is the only available sample

Table 4.4 Non-epithelial malignant tumors that may express panCK

Tumor type	panCK (%)
Epithelioid morphology	
Melanoma (skin, soft tissue)	10 %
Mesothelioma	95 %
Epithelioid angiosarcoma	65 %
Epithelioid hemangioendothelioma	15 %
Epithelioid leiomyosarcoma	10 %
Epithelioid MPNST	20 %
Epithelioid rhabdomyosarcoma	25 %
Epithelioid sarcoma	80 %
Osteosarcoma	<10 %
Alveolar soft part sarcoma	None
Synovial sarcoma	65 %
Chordoma	100 %
Epithelioid GIST	Rare
Paraganglioma	<10 %
Seminoma	30 %
Large cell lymphoma	Rare
Plasma cell neoplasms	20 %
Others	
DPSRCT	90 %
Ewing sarcoma/PNET	15 %

Abbreviations of tumor entities: *DPSRCT* desmoplastic small round cell tumor, *GIST* gastrointestinal stromal tumor, *MPNST* malignant peripheral nerve sheath tumor, *PNET* primitive neuroectodermal tumor

type for staining, nuclear markers such as SOX10 and MITF are preferred; both stain the epithelioid and spindle variant of melanoma with high sensitivity (Figs. 4.9 and 4.10).

Hematopoietic Markers

CD45 is highly specific for hematopoietic cells. However, a few hematopoietic neoplasms might be negative for CD45, including anaplastic large cell lymphoma, lymphoblastic lymphoma,

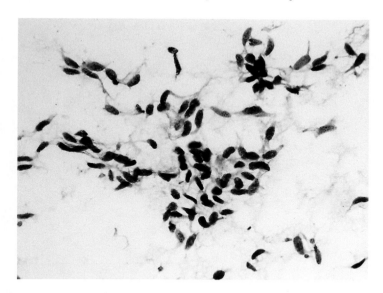

Fig. 4.9 Immunostaining using direct smear when cell block is not available (example 7): positive SOX10 staining on a smear confirms a metastatic melanoma with spindle cell features (SOX10 stain)

myeloid sarcoma, plasma cell neoplasms, Reed–Sternberg cells and variants in classical Hodgkin lymphoma, and follicular dendritic cell sarcoma (Table 4.5). In these circumstances, CD43 should be used to increase the detectability when these tumors are in the differential diagnosis.

Flow cytometric immunophenotyping is critical for subtyping B-cell lymphoma. When it is not available, cytospin or direct smears can be used for immunostaining, such as kappa and lambda, CD20, and CD3 (Figs. 4.11 and 4.12). Ki67 staining to assess tumor proliferation is an important part of a lymphoma workup because it helps grading of non-Hodgkin B-cell lymphomas (Fig. 4.13). SOX11 is highly sensitive and specific for mantle cell lymphoma; it can be used as an adjunct to immunophenotyping to increase the diagnostic certainty in a primary diagnostic setting or

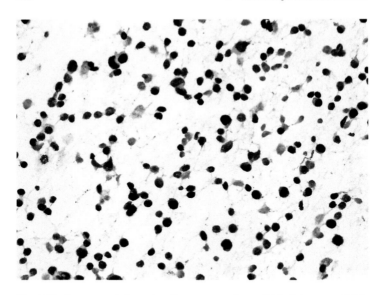

Fig. 4.10 Immunostaining using direct smear when cell block is not available (example 8): positive MITF staining on a smear confirms a metastatic melanoma in the parotid gland (MITF stain)

Table 4.5 Hematopoietic neoplasms that may be negative for CD45

Tumor	CD45 (%)
Anaplastic large cell lymphoma	50–80
Classical Hodgkin lymphoma (Reed–Sternberg cell/variants)	0–10
Follicular dendritic cell sarcoma	0
Lymphoblastic lymphoma	25–50
Myeloid sarcoma	50–80
Plasma cell neoplasms	65

as a sole diagnostic marker to confirm mantle cell lymphoma in a recurrent setting, especially when a patient has a known history of MCL and the FNA sample has insufficient cells for flow cytometric immunophenotyping (Fig. 4.14).

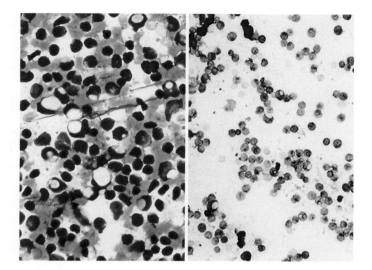

Fig. 4.11 Immunostaining using direct smear when cell block is not available (example 9): positive CD20 staining on a cytospin slide supports B-cell lineage of a lymphoma with signet ring cell features (*left*, Diff-Quik stain; *right*, CD20 stain)

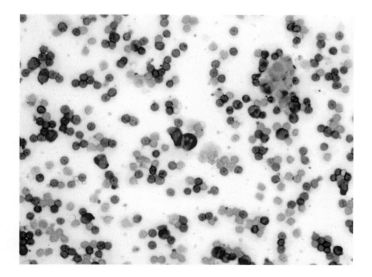

Fig. 4.12 Immunostaining using direct smear when cell block is not available (example 10): positive CD3 staining on a cytospin supports T-cell lineage of a peripheral T-cell lymphoma (CD3 stain)

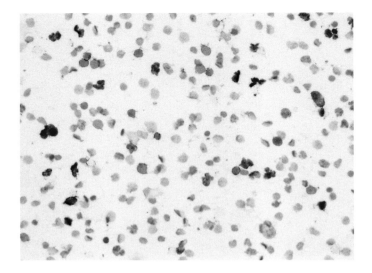

Fig. 4.13 Immunostaining using direct smear when cell block is not available (example 11): Ki-67 staining on a cytospin helps grading B-cell lymphoma, especially in documenting a possible transformation of low-grade lymphoma to higher-grade form (Ki67 stain)

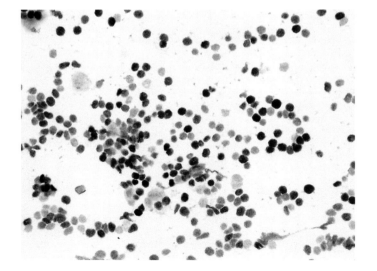

Fig. 4.14 Immunostaining using direct smear when cell block is not available (example 12): positive SOX11 on a smear helps confirmation of mantle cell lymphoma (SOX11)

Mesenchymal Markers

Vimentin is often considered to as a mesenchymal marker because nearly all types of sarcomas express this marker except for rare entities such as alveolar soft part sarcoma. Vimentin is sometimes used to differentiate sarcoma from carcinoma (mostly vimentin negative). However, vimentin is a nonspecific marker for recognizing sarcomas because it can be variably expressed in tumors of other lineages, including some carcinomas, lymphomas, melanoma, mesothelioma, and germ cell tumors (Table 4.6). Additional specific markers are often needed for further classification (Figs. 4.15 and 4.16).

Desmin is commonly used as a first-line marker to screen for myogenic differentiation. However, non-myogenic tumors may unexpectedly express desmin, including desmoplastic small round cell tumor, blastemal component of Wilms tumor, and mesothelial cells (benign > malignant). However, these entities are negative for muscle-specific actin or smooth muscle actin. Therefore, desmin should be used together with actins in some cases.

Determination of Tumor Subtype and Possible Origin (Step 2) (Figs. 1.9 and 4.8)

Of the four broad categories of malignancy, carcinoma is the most common. The major subtypes of carcinoma include adenocarcinoma, squamous carcinoma, neuroendocrine carcinoma, and others such as urothelial carcinoma, renal cell carcinoma, hepatocellular carcinoma, and adrenal cortical carcinoma. The cytologic features of these subtypes are outlined in Chap. 3.

Of the abovementioned subtypes, adenocarcinoma is the most commonly encountered. MOC31, BerEP4, and B72.3 are markers of adenocarcinoma in general; however, they are usually used in effusion samples to distinguish adenocarcinoma (positive) from mesothelial hyperplasia or mesothelioma (negative). The com-

Table 4.6 Positive vimentin expression in non-mesenchymal tumors

Epithelial lineage
Adrenal cortical carcinoma
Breast carcinoma including metaplastic type
Endometrial adenocarcinoma
Myoepithelial carcinoma
Ovarian serous carcinoma
Renal cell carcinoma
Spindle cell/sarcomatoid carcinoma of various sites
Thyroid carcinoma including anaplastic type
Salivary duct carcinoma
Small cell carcinoma
Other lineages
Lymphoma (especially B-lymphoblastic and large cell lymphoma)
Melanoma
Mesothelioma
Seminoma, yolk sac tumor

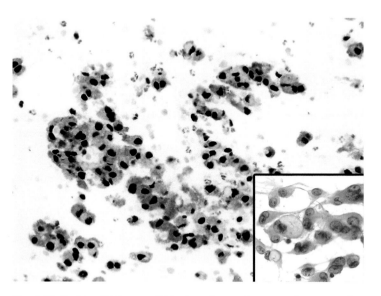

Fig. 4.15 Positive ERG on a cell block section confirms vascular nature of an epithelioid hemangioendothelioma (ERG stain; *inset*, Papanicolaou stain)

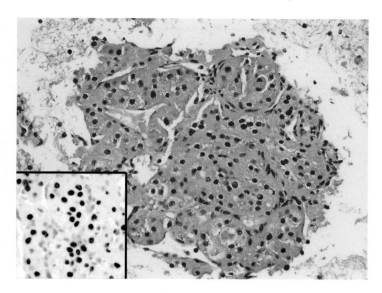

Fig. 4.16 Positive TFE3 on a cell block section confirms a diagnosis of alveolar soft part sarcoma (H&E-stained cell block; *inset*: TFE3 stain)

mon second-tier immunomarkers are CK7 and CK20 panel (Table 4.7) to define possible primary origins. Adenocarcinoma with a CK7-negative and CK20-positive expression pattern is quite specific for colorectal origin. However, adenocarcinoma of many organ sites is CK7-positive/CK20-negative; adenocarcinoma of the pancreaticobiliary tract, stomach, and esophagus show variable CK7 and CK20 expression patterns. In most cases, CK7, with or without CK20, is ordered together with one or more specific markers (see section "Determination of Primary Origin") for working up an adenocarcinoma.

For squamous carcinoma, the general markers include P40, P63, and CK5/6. There is virtually no site-specific marker for squamous carcinoma; however, P16 immunostaining, together with HPV testing using in situ hybridization (ISH), can help determine the possible site because HPV-associated squamous carcinoma

Table 4.7 Common CK7 and CK20 staining patterns in tumors from various primary sites

CK7 and CK20 expression	Tumor and origin
CK7+/CK20−	Lung: non-small cell carcinoma, adenocarcinoma
	Breast: ductal carcinoma, lobular carcinoma
	Endometrium: adenocarcinoma
	Endocervix: adenocarcinoma
	Ovary: adenocarcinoma (nonmucinous)
	Kidney: renal cell carcinoma (papillary, chromophobe, collecting duct and medullary)
	Thyroid carcinoma (papillary, follicular, medullary)
	Thymus: thymic carcinoma
	Salivary gland: ductal carcinoma
	Mesothelium: mesothelioma
	Uterine cervix: squamous carcinoma
CK7−/CK20+	Colon and rectum: adenocarcinoma
	Skin: Merkel cell carcinoma
	Salivary gland: small cell carcinoma
CK7+/CK20+	Genitourinary tract: urothelial carcinoma (may also CK7+/CK20−)
	Ovary: mucinous adenocarcinoma
	Stomach and esophagus: adenocarcinoma
	Pancreatic/biliary tract: adenocarcinoma including cholangiocarcinoma
CK7−/CK20−	Liver: hepatocellular carcinoma
	Kidney: renal cell carcinoma (clear cell)
	Prostate: adenocarcinoma
	Adrenal gland: adrenal cortical carcinoma
	Lung: small cell carcinoma
	Gastrointestinal tract and lung: carcinoid tumor
	Gonadal or extragonadal sites: germ cell tumors
	Head and neck, esophagus, lung: squamous carcinoma

−, <10 % of cases are positive; −/+, 10–50 % of cases are positive; +/−, 50–70 % of cases are positive; +, >70 of cases are positive

1) Medullary carcinoma of the colon is CK7−/CK20−
2) Adenocarcinomas of the pancreaticobiliary tract, stomach, and esophagus show variable CK7/CK20 patterns
3) Neuroendocrine carcinomas of the lung, liver, and small bowel are either CK7+/CK20− or CK7−/CK20−. Carcinoid tumors of the gastrointestinal tract and lung are mostly CK7−/CK20−

usually occurs in the uterine cervix and anogenital and oropharyngeal sites. Squamous carcinoma of the head and neck, esophagus, and lungs is mostly negative for both CK7 and CK20, whereas squamous carcinoma of the cervix is often positive for CK7 but negative for CK20 (Table 4.7).

The general markers for neuroendocrine carcinoma include chromogranin, synaptophysin, and CD56. Like squamous carcinoma, there are no reliable site-specific markers for neuroendocrine carcinoma. Neuroendocrine carcinomas of the lungs, liver, and small bowel are either CK7-positive/CK20-negative or negative for both markers; carcinoid tumors of the gastrointestinal tract and lungs are mostly negative for both markers (Table 4.7). With the development and increasing use of new markers, some have been found to be "unexpected" neuroendocrine markers. These include TTF1, CDX2, SATB2, PR, PAX8 (Table 4.1), and CDH17 (Table 4.2). TTF1 positivity is more common in neuroendocrine tumors of the lungs than in those of other origins; expression of PAX8 and PR is reportedly supportive of pancreatic origin. With variable frequencies, CDH17 labels neuroendocrine tumors of the pancreas and entire gastrointestinal tract; CDX2 labels neuroendocrine tumors of the small and large intestines, and SATB2 positivity is usually confined to neuroendocrine tumors of the left colon and rectum. Traps and tips are further discussed in section "Neuroendocrine Tumors and Differential Diagnosis".

Urothelial carcinoma is usually positive for both CK7 and CK20, with a small subset of cases being CK7-positive but CK20-negative. Renal cell carcinoma, hepatocellular carcinoma, and adrenal cortical carcinoma are typically negative for both markers (Table 4.7). Their specific diagnostic panels are listed in Table 4.8.

Typically, mesothelioma is positive for CK7 and negative for CK20, and germ cell tumors and chordoma are negative for both markers. Their specific immunophenotypic features are covered in Tables 4.9 and 4.11 (Figs. 3.30, 4.17, and 4.18).

Table 4.8 Confirmatory markers for carcinomas from various primary sites

Tumor and origin	Confirmatory if positive	Others
Adrenal cortical CA	Melan A (clone A103), inhibin, calretinin, SF1, synaptophysin	panCK−/+, EMA−, chromogranin−
Breast CA	ER, GATA3, GCDFP15, mammaglobin for AdCA CK903, P63 for metaplastic CA	
Endocervical AdCA	PAX8, P16 (strong and diffuse), HPV in situ	CEA+, ER−/+, vimentin−
Endometrial AdCA	PAX8, ER	Vimentin+, CEA−/+, PAX2−/+, P16−/+, HPV−
GI tract AdCA, upper and pancreas	CK7, CDH17, CDX2	
GI tract AdCA, lower	CK20, CDX2, SATB2, CDH17	Villin+
Hepatocellular CA	Arginase, HepPar1, Glypican3, polyclonal CEA and CD10 (canalicular pattern), AFP	panCK+/−, CAM5.2+
Lung AdCA	TTF1, Napsin A	Surfactant+/−
Merkel cell CA, skin	panCK, CK20 (perinuclear dot pattern), chromogranin, synaptophysin, neurofilament, MCPyV	See Table 4.15
Neuroendocrine CA, various sites	Chromogranin, synaptophysin, CD56	TTF1+/−, CDX2+/− (see Table 4.12)
Ovarian/primary peritoneal serous CA	PAX8, WT1, ER	
Ovarian clear cellCA	PAX8	

Pheochromocytoma, paraganglioma	Chromogranin, synaptophysin	panCK–/+, inhibin–, Melan A (clone A103)–
Prostate AdCA	PSA, PAP, NKX3.1, prostein	ERG+/–
Renal cell CA	PAX8, RCC, CD10, CAIX, AMACR	See Tables 4.17 and 4.18
Salivary ductal CA	GCDFP15, androgen receptor	GATA3+/–
Small cell CA, various sites	Chromogranin, synaptophysin, CD56, TTF1	See Table 4.15
Squamous CA, various sites	P40, P63, CK5/6, CK903 (HPV in situ and P16 staining for cervix, anogenital and oropharyngeal origins)	
Thymic CA	CD5, P63, PAX8	CD117
Thyroid CA, papillary or follicular	TTF1, PAX8, thyroglobulin	See Table 4.16
Thyroid CA, medullary	Calcitonin, TTF1, CEA, chromogranin, synaptophysin	PAX8–/+ (see Table 4.16)
Thyroid CA, anaplastic	PAX8	TTF1–/+, thyroglobulin– (see Table 4.16)
Urothelial CA	GATA3, uroplakin, CK903, P63, CK5/6, thrombomodulin, P40, CK20	

–, <10 % of cases are positive; –/+, 10–50 % of cases are positive; +/–, 50–70 % of cases are positive; +, >70 of cases are positive

Abbreviations: *AdCA* adenocarcinoma, *CA* carcinoma

Table 4.9 Confirmatory markers for melanoma and other tumor types

Tumor type and origin	Confirmatory if positive	Others
Melanoma, skin or soft tissue	Melan A/MART1, SOX10, MITF, S100, HMB45, tyrosinase	See Table 4.15
Mesothelioma, serous cavity	Calretinin, CK5/6, WT1, D2-40	MOC31−, BerEP4−
Germ cell tumors, gonadal or extragonadal sites	Sall4, PLAP, OCT3/4, CD117, Glypican3, CD30, AFP, NANOG	panCK+/−; see Table 4.19
Sex cord stromal tumors, gonad	SF1, inhibin, calretinin, Melan A (clone A103)	panCK−/+

−, <10 % of cases are positive; −/+, 10–50 % of cases are positive; +/−, 50–70 % of cases are positive; +, >70 of cases are positive

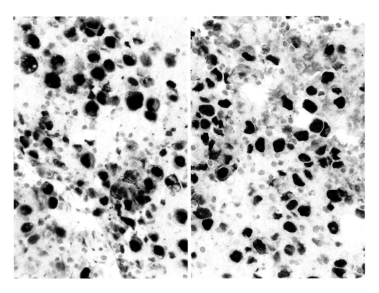

Fig. 4.17 Positive OCT3/4 (*left*) staining and Sall4 (*right*) staining on cell block sections confirm a diagnosis of seminoma

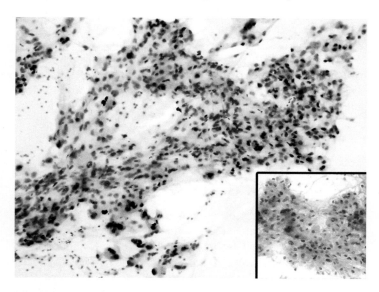

Fig. 4.18 Immunostaining using direct smear when cell block is not available (example 13): positive brachyury staining on a smear confirms a diagnosis of chordoma (brachyury stain; *inset*, Papanicolaou stain)

Determination of Specific Primary Origin (Step 3) (Figs. 1.9 and 4.8)

In most circumstances, the CK7 and CK20 expression panel is insufficient to pinpoint the primary origin of an adenocarcinoma except for colorectal adenocarcinoma. Therefore, third-tier immunomarkers are needed.

Table 4.8 lists the confirmatory markers for carcinomas from various organ sites.

Table 4.9 lists the confirmatory markers for melanoma (from skin or soft tissue), mesothelioma (from the serous cavity), germ cell tumors (from gonadal or extragonadal sites), and sex cord stromal tumors (from the gonads). Of note, Melan A/MART1, SOX10, MITF, S100, and HMB45 are quite specific for melanoma and its soft tissue counterpart. Most of these markers are also present in other melanosome-containing tumors, such as melanotic nerve sheath tumors and PEComas (encompassing angiomyolipoma, clear cell sugar tumor, and lymphangioleiomyomatosis) (Tables 4.1 and 4.2).

Table 4.10 lists the confirmatory markers for hematopoietic malignancies that are often encountered.

Table 4.11 lists the confirmatory markers for mesenchymal malignancies from soft tissue and bone.

Neuroendocrine Tumors and Differential Diagnosis (Table 4.12)

Neuroendocrine tumors are composed of two categories: epithelial (e.g., carcinoid, pancreatic endocrine tumor, medullary thyroid carcinoma, Merkel cell carcinoma, and small cell carcinoma) and non-epithelial (e.g., neuroblastoma, pheochromocytoma/paraganglioma). Epithelial neuroendocrine tumors are positive for panCK, with the exception of small cell carcinoma, which shows variable reactivity, whereas non-epithelial neuroendocrine tumors are negative for panCK. PanCK staining in small cell carcinoma and Merkel cell carcinoma has a perinuclear dot-like pattern, as does CK20 in Merkel cell carcinoma.

The general cytologic features of neuroendocrine tumors are outlined in Chap. 3. The important clue is finely stippled ("salt and pepper") chromatin and inconspicuous nucleoli. Chromogranin and synaptophysin are the first-line screening markers for neuroendocrine differentiation with synaptophysin being more sensitive and chromogranin being more specific (Fig. 4.19). Generally, chromogranin and synaptophysin are sufficient to identify most neuroendocrine tumors, especially low-grade ones. CD56 is a neuroendocrine marker that is generally more sensitive than are chromogranin and synaptophysin, but it is not routinely used as a screening marker since it is less specific. For example, CD56 can label synovial sarcoma, steroid-producing tumors, sex core stromal tumors, peripheral nerve sheath tumors, rhabdomyosarcoma, and several lymphomas and plasma cell neoplasms. However, CD56 can be saved for cases that are suspicious for high-grade neuroendocrine tumors (especially small cell carcinoma) but show a negative reaction to the two first-line markers.

Table 4.10 Confirmatory markers for hematopoietic malignancies

Tumor type	Confirmatory if positive	Others
Anaplastic large cell lymphoma	CD45/CD43, CD30, ALK1, EMA	CD15-, PAX5-
Hodgkin lymphoma, classical (Reed–Sternberg cells/variants)	CD15, CD30, PAX5 (weak)	Fascin+/-, CD45-, EMA-, CD20-/+, OCT2-/+, BOB1-/+
Hodgkin lymphoma, nodular lymphocyte predominant (popcorn cells)	CD45, CD20, PAX5 (strong)	CD15-, CD30-, OCT2+, BOB1+
Non-Hodgkin lymphoma, B cell	CD45, CD79a, CD19, CD20, PAX5	See Table 5.1
Non-Hodgkin lymphoma, T cell	CD45, CD3, CD5, CD7	
Lymphoblastic lymphoma	CD45/CD43, TdT, CD34, B-cell markers (PAX5, CD79a), or T-cell marker (CD3)	See Table 4.15
Plasma cell neoplasms	CD45/CD43, CD38, CD138, cytoplasmic kappa or lambda, CD79a	CD20-, CD19-, MUM1+/-
Myeloid sarcoma (granulocytic sarcoma)	CD45/CD43, CD34, CD117, myeloperoxidase, CD33, CD15, CD13	TdT-/+
Langerhans cell histiocytosis	CD1a, S100	CD45 + (weak)
Follicular dendritic cell sarcoma	Clusterin, Fascin, CD21, CD23, CD35	CD45-, S100-/+
Interdigitating dendritic cell sarcoma	S100, Fascin	CD45 weak+/-, CD21-, CD23-, CD35-, Clusterin-

-, <10 % of cases are positive; -/+, 10–50 % of cases are positive; +/-, 50–70 % of cases are positive; +, >70 % of cases are positive

Table 4.11 Confirmatory markers for mesenchymal malignancies from soft tissue and bone

Tumor type	Confirmatory if positive	Others
Alveolar soft part sarcoma	TFE3, Cathepsin-K	S100−/+, CD34−/+, CD117−/+, vimentin−
Angiosarcoma	ERG, CD31, Factor VIII, FLI1, CD34	Kaposi sarcoma is also HHV8+
Chordoma	Brachyury, CK, EMA, S100	See Table 4.15
DPSRCT	CK, desmin, WT1, CD56	Smooth muscle markers+/−
Endometrial stromal sarcoma	CD10, ER	ERG−/+, CD31−
Epithelioid sarcoma	CK, CD34, loss of INI1	See Table 4.15
Ewing sarcoma/PNET	NKX2.2, CD99 (diffuse membranous), FLI1	
GIST	CD117, DOG1, CD34	Smooth muscle markers+/−
Inflammatory myofibroblastic tumor	ALK (cytoplasmic)	Patchy CK+ in epithelioid variant
Leiomyosarcoma	SMA, desmin, caldesmon	S100−/+
Liposarcoma, well-differentiated and dedifferentiated types	MDM2 and CDK4	
Liposarcoma, myxoid/round cell	NY-ESO-1	
MPNST	S100	SOX10−/+, negative for other melanoma markers, CK+/− in epithelioid variant
Rhabdomyosarcoma	Desmin, myogenin, MyoD1	Patchy CK+ in epithelioid variant
Solitary fibrous tumor	STAT6, BCL2, CD34	CD99+
Synovial sarcoma	TLE1, CK(+/−)	See Tables 4.14 and 4.15
Paraganglioma/pheochromocytoma	Chromogranin, synaptophysin	See Table 4.12
PEComas	MART1, HMB45, MITF, SMA, desmin, Cathepsin-K	

−, <10 % of cases are positive; −/+, 10–50 % of cases are positive; +/−, 50–70 % of cases are positive; +, >70 of cases are positive
Abbreviation of tumor entities: *DPSRCT* desmoplastic small round cell tumor, *GIST* gastrointestinal stromal tumor, *MPNST* malignant peripheral nerve sheath tumor, *PEComas* perivascular epithelioid cell neoplasms (including angiomyolipoma, clear cell sugar tumor, lymphangioleio-

Table 4.12 Differential diagnosis of neuroendocrine tumors

Tumor type	PanCK	Chromogranin	Synaptophysin	Others
Carcinoid tumor	+	+	+	TTF1+ in the lung, CDX2+ in the GI tract
Medullary thyroid carcinoma	+	+	+	Calcitonin+, CEA+, TTF1+
Merkel cell carcinoma	+	+	+	CK20 and CK: perinuclear dot pattern, neurofilament+, MCPyV
Pancreatic endocrine tumor	+	+	+	Beware of synaptophysin+ in solid pseudopapillary tumor
Parathyroid tumor	+	+	+	PTH+
Small cell carcinoma	+/−	+/−	+	TTF1+ in the lung and +/−in other sites; use CD56 if other neuroendocrine markers are negative
Neuroblastoma	−	+	+	
Pheochromocytoma/paraganglioma	−	+	+	S100 in sustentacular cells

−, <10 % of cases are positive; −/+, 10–50 % of cases are positive; +/−, 50–70 % of cases are positive; +, >70 % of cases are positive

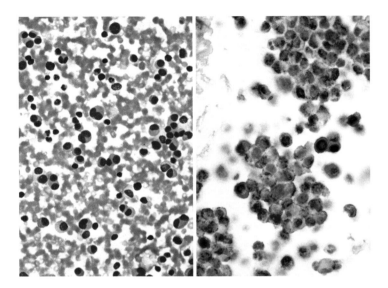

Fig. 4.19 Immunostaining using direct smear when cell block is not available (example 14): positive chromogranin staining confirms a diagnosis of metastatic neuroendocrine carcinoma with plasmacytoid features in a lumbar vertebral bone and excludes a differential diagnosis of plasma cell neoplasm (*left*, Diff-Quik stain; *right*, chromogranin stain)

Caution should be taken not to use synaptophysin alone because a few non-neuroendocrine tumors can be positive for synaptophysin but not for chromogranin. These include adrenal cortical tumors, pancreatic solid pseudopapillary tumor, desmoplastic small round cell tumors, thymic carcinoma, and thyroid non-medullary carcinomas.

In pancreatic tumors, low-grade pancreatic endocrine tumor (i.e., islet cell tumor), solid pseudopapillary tumor, and acinar cell carcinoma can show significant overlap in their cytologic features, and immunostaining workup is often required for a differential diagnosis (Table 4.13). A common mistake is to use synaptophysin as the sole marker for confirming the neuroendocrine nature of a case in which only one slide is available for staining. Solid pseudopapillary tumor can be positive for this marker, leading to a misdiagnosis of a pancreatic endocrine carcinoma, especially if the clinical presentation is not typical (Fig. 4.20). Therefore, synaptophysin should

Table 4.13 Differential diagnosis of pancreatic endocrine tumor, solid pseudopapillary tumor, and acinar cell carcinoma

Marker	Pancreatic endocrine tumor	Acinar cell carcinoma	Solid pseudopapillary tumor
panCK	+	+	−/+
CD56	+	−/+	+/−
Synaptophysin	+	−/+	+/−
Chromogranin	+	−/+	−
CD10	−	−	+
nuclear β-catenin	−	−/+	+
Trypsin	−	+	−/+
PR	+/−	−	+
Vimentin	−	−	+

−, <10 % of cases are positive; −/+, 10–50 % of cases are positive; +/−, 50–70 % of cases are positive; +, >70 of cases are positive

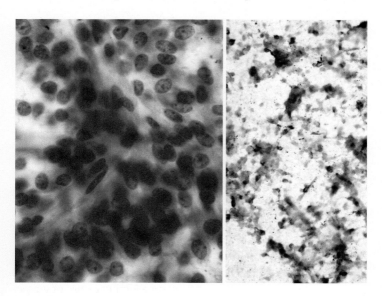

Fig. 4.20 An example of diagnostic traps: using synaptophysin as a sole marker to confirm neuroendocrine nature of a tumor is not reliable. A single synaptophysin positivity on a smear of a pancreatic lesion from a 46-year-old man was thought to support pancreatic endocrine tumor. A subsequent surgical resection proved to be a solid pseudopapillary tumor of the pancreas (*left*, Papanicolaou stain; *right*, synaptophysin)

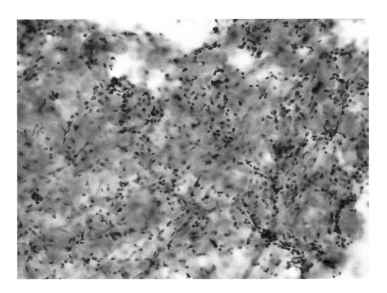

Fig. 4.21 Amyloid material in a pancreatic lesion is an important clue of pancreatic endocrine tumor. It may be overlooked or misinterpreted as nonspecific fibrous tissue in the background (Papanicolaou stain)

not be used as a sole marker to confirm a neuroendocrine nature. Amyloid material, if found, is supportive of a neuroendocrine carcinoma (Figs. 4.21 and 4.22).

The unexpected neuroendocrine markers, such as TTF1, CDX2, SATB2, PR, PAX8, and CDH17, have been discussed in section "Determination of Tumor Subtype and Possible Origin" and listed in Tables 4.1 and 4.2.

Spindle Cell Malignancies and Differential Diagnosis (Table 4.14)

Malignant tumors with spindle cell features are listed in section "Tumors with Spindle Cell Appearance" in Chap. 3 and Fig. 1.10 and illustrated in Figs. 2.12 and 3.42–3.51. The general cytologic features of sarcoma, the most common entity in this group, are

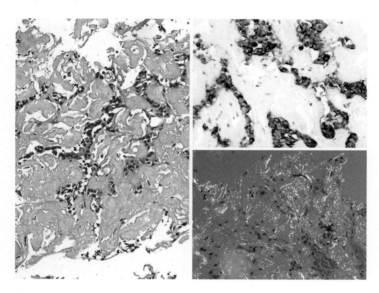

Fig. 4.22 Amyloid material on cell block section showing homogenous and amorphous extracellular material (*left*), which shows characteristic apple-green birefringence with polarized light microscopy (*right lower*). This tumor was strongly positive for chromogranin (*right upper*)

described in Chap. 2. Of the spindle cell carcinomas or sarcomatoid carcinomas, those commonly seen in cytology practice are from genitourinary sites (e.g., renal cell carcinoma and urothelial carcinoma), the lungs (e.g., squamous carcinoma), and the breasts (e.g., metaplastic carcinoma). The characteristic immunostaining profile of each entity is listed in Table 4.14.

Small Round Blue Cell Tumors and Differential Diagnosis (Table 4.15)

Tumors with small blue cell features are listed in section "Tumors with Small Cell Appearance" in Chap. 3 and Fig. 1.10 and illustrated in Figs. 2.4, 2.5, 3.25, and 3.52–3.58. The general cytologic

Table 4.14 Differential diagnosis of malignant tumors with spindle cell morphology

Tumor type	Tumor/origin	Positive	Negative
Sarcoma	Leiomyosarcoma	Desmin, MSA, SMA	
	Rhabdomyosarcoma	Desmin, MSA, myogenin, MyoD1	SMA, CK
	Angiosarcoma	CD31, CD34, Factor VIII, ERG, FLI1, Ulex1	Desmin, MSA
	MPNST	S100, CD34	Desmin, MSA
	Dedifferentiated liposarcoma	MDM2 and CDK4, S100	Desmin, MSA
	Malignant fibrous histiocytoma	CD68(+/−)	Desmin, MSA
Spindle cell carcinoma	Lung	CK, P40, P63, CK5/6, CK903	
	Kidney	CK, PAX8, CAIX, RCC, CD10	See Tables 4.17 and 4.18
	Urothelial cell	CK, GATA3, thrombomodulin, uroplakin, CK903, P63	
	Breast	CK, GATA3, mammaglobin, CK903, P63	
Spindle cell melanoma		MART1, SOX10, S100, MITF, tyrosinase	CK
Lymphoma, sclerosing large cell		CD45, CD20, PAX5, CD79a	
Others	GIST	CD117, DOG1, CD34(+/−)	CK, SMA(−/+)
	Synovial sarcoma	TLE1, CK	CD34, desmin, MSA

−, <10 % of cases are positive; −/+, 10–50 % of cases are positive; +/−, 50–70 % of cases are positive; +, >70 % of cases are positive
Abbreviations of tumor entities: *GIST* gastrointestinal stromal tumor, *MPNST* malignant peripheral nerve sheath tumor

features of small cell carcinoma, Merkel cell carcinoma, melanoma, and lymphoma are described in Chap. 2 and section "Neuroendocrine Carcinoma" in Chap. 3. The characteristic immunostaining profile of each entity is listed in Table 4.15.

It is of note that, in certain clinical contexts, differential diagnosis should include poorly differentiated or basaloid squamous carcinoma, the solid component of adenoid cystic carcinoma, metastatic basal cell carcinoma, and granulosa cell tumor (Figs. 3.59–3.62).

Differential Diagnosis of Thyroid Carcinomas

Different subtypes of thyroid carcinomas are illustrated in Figs. 1.8, 3.8, 3.9, 3.14, 3.24, 3.46, 3.63, 3.72, and 3.97. The characteristic immunostaining profile of each subtype is listed in Table 4.16.

Differential Diagnosis of Kidney Tumors

The general cytologic features of renal cell carcinomas are described in 3.1.4 and illustrated in Figs. 1.5, 3.27, 3.69, and 3.75. The characteristic immunostaining profile of each subtype and differential diagnosis are listed in Tables 4.17 and 4.18.

Differential Diagnosis of Germ Cell Tumors

The general cytologic features of seminoma/dysgerminoma are described in section "Germ Cell Tumors" in Chap. 3 and illustrated in Figs. 3.31, 3.41, 3.79, and 4.17. The characteristic immunostaining profile of each subtype of germ cell tumors is listed in Table 4.19.

Table 4.15 Differential diagnosis of small round blue cell tumors

Tumor type	Positive	Negative	Cytogenetic changes
Small cell carcinoma	CK(+/−), synaptophysin, chromogranin, CD56, TTF1	CD45	
Merkel cell carcinoma	CK, CK20, synaptophysin, chromogranin, neurofilament, MCPyV	TTF1, CD45	
Ewing sarcoma/PNET	NKX2.2, CD99 (diffuse membranous), FLI1	CD45, chromogranin, TLE1, CK(−/+), synaptophysin(−/+)	See Table 6.1
Synovial sarcoma	TLE1, CK, CD99	CD34, desmin	See Table 6.1
Rhabdomyosarcoma	Myogenin, MyoD1, desmin	CK(−/+), CD45	See Table 6.1
Small cell osteosarcoma	Vimentin, CD99		
Non-Hodgkin lymphoma	CD45, B-cell (CD20, CD79a, PAX5), or T-cell (CD3) markers	CK	See Table 5.1
Lymphoblastic lymphoma	CD45(+/−), TdT, CD34, CD10, B cell markers (PAX5, CD79a) or T cell markers (CD3), CD99, FLI1	CK	
Melanoma	Melan A/MART1, HMB45, S100, SOX10, MITF	CK, CD45	
Neuroblastoma	Synaptophysin, chromogranin	CK, CD99	Hyperdiploidy, 1p deletion

Wilms tumor (blastemal component predominant)	WT1, desmin	CD45, CD99(−/+)	See Table 6.1
DPSRCT	CK, desmin, WT1, CD56, CD99(−/+)	CD45, SMA(−/+) synaptophysin(−/+)	See Table 6.1
Mesenchymal chondrosarcoma	SOX9		

−, <10 % of cases are positive; −/+, 10–50 % of cases are positive; +/−, 50–70 % of cases are positive; +, >70 of cases are positive

Abbreviation of tumor entities: *DPSRCT* desmoplastic small round cell tumor, *PNET* primitive neuroectodermal tumor

1) TTF1 in small cell carcinoma of the lung is mostly (90 %) positive; its expression in small cell carcinoma of non-lung origins (prostate, bladder, cervix, etc.) is less frequent

2) CD99 should be diffuse membranous staining in Ewing sarcoma. DPSRCT usually shows cytoplasmic CD99

Table 4.16 Differential diagnosis of thyroid carcinomas

Marker	Papillary thyroid carcinoma	Thyroid follicular carcinoma	Thyroid medullary carcinoma	Anaplastic thyroid carcinoma
Thyroglobulin	+	+	−	−
TTF1	+	+	+	−/+
PAX8	+	+	−/+	+/−
Chromogranin, synaptophysin	−	−	+	−
CEA	−	−	+	−
Calcitonin	−	−	+	−

−, <10 % of cases are positive; −/+, 10–50 % of cases are positive; +/−, 50–70 % of cases are positive; +, >70 of cases are positive

Cancer of Unknown Primary Origin (CUP)

CUP is a heterogeneous group of cancers defined by the presence of metastatic disease with no identified primary tumor after an "adequate" diagnostic workup. The primary origin of some CUPs may be identified only at autopsy. Approximately 3–5 % of new malignant diagnoses are classified as CUP. Because of the lack of effective therapeutic regimens, patients usually receive broad-spectrum empiric chemotherapy and most of these patients have a poor prognosis. Currently, there is poor consensus on the extent of diagnostic and pathologic evaluations necessary. However, with the availability of sophisticated imaging techniques and after an extensive multidisciplinary workup, a true CUP is virtually rare.

The most common sites of involvement are lymph nodes, liver, bones, and lungs. The most common sites of origin (if discovered) are the lung, pancreaticobiliarytract, kidney or adrenal gland, large bowel, stomach, and genital system. CUP theoretically includes all types of malignancies (i.e., carcinomas, melanoma, lymphomas, and sarcomas). However, the vast majority of CUP cases are carcinomas, of which adenocarcinoma is the most common, followed by squamous carcinoma and neuroendocrine carcinoma. Among the non-epithelial malignant tumors, CUP is more often seen in melanoma than tumors with other lineages.

Table 4.17 Differential diagnosis of kidney tumors

Tumor type	Positive	Negative
Clear cell renal cell carcinoma	PAX8, CAIX (diffuse membranous), CD10, RCC, EMA, vimentin	AMACR(−/+), CK7(−/+)
Papillary renal cell carcinoma	PAX8, AMACR, CK7, RCC, CD10(+/−)	CAIX(−/+)
Clear cell papillary renal cell carcinoma	PAX8, CAIX (cuplike), CK7	AMACR, CD10(−/+)
Xp11 translocation renal cell carcinoma	PAX8(+/−), TFE3, AMACR, Cathepsin-K(+/−)	panCK, EMA, CK7, CAIX(−/+), HMB45(−/+), MART1(−/+)
t(6;11) renal cell carcinoma	PAX8(+/−), TFEB, Cathepsin-K, HMB45, MART1	CK7, panCK(−/+), EMA(−/+), CAIX(−/+)
Chromophobe renal cell carcinoma	PAX8, CD117, CK7, Ksp-cadherin	CAIX, vimentin, AMACR(−/+), CD10(−/+)
Oncocytoma	PAX8, CD117, Ksp-cadherin	CAIX, vimentin, CK7(−/+), AMACR(−/+)
Epithelioid angiomyolipoma	Cathepsin-K, HMB45, MART1, SMA, desmin	panCK, PAX8, EMA, CAIX

−, <10 % of cases are positive; −/+, 10–50 % of cases are positive; +/−, 50–70 % of cases are positive; +, >70 of cases are positive

1) CD10 and RCC markers both have low sensitivity and specificity for renal cell carcinoma

2) CAIX positivity is very sensitive and specific for clear cell renal cell carcinoma and requires diffuse and membranous staining pattern; it is cuplike membranous staining pattern in clear cell papillary renal cell carcinoma. Nonspecific CAIX staining may be seen in various tumors adjacent to areas of necrosis or focal cytoplasmic staining in high-grade areas because of hypoxia/ischemia

3) All are positive for EMA except for translocation renal cell carcinoma, which can be used to confirm epithelial/carcinoma nature for rare CK-negative renal cell carcinoma and distinguish renal cell carcinoma from adrenal cortical tumors (EMA negative)

4) All are positive for vimentin except for chromophobe and oncocytoma

5) Two benign tumors, oncocytoma and angiomyolipoma, are included in the table for differential diagnosis

Table 4.18 Differential diagnosis of kidney tumors with positive CK7 staining and high-grade cytologic features

Tumor type	Positive	Negative
Collecting duct carcinoma	PAX8, CK7, INI1(+/−)	GATA3, P63
Medullary carcinoma	PAX8, CK7, OCT4(+/−)	INI1, P63
Upper tract urothelial carcinoma	GATA3, CK7, P63, CK903, thrombomodulin, uroplakin, INI1, CAIX(+/−)	PAX8(−/+), AMACR(−/+)

−, <10 % of cases are positive; −/+, 10–50 % of cases are positive; +/−, 50–70 % of cases are positive; +, >70 of cases are positive

Table 4.19 Differential diagnosis of germ cell tumors

Tumor type	Positive	Negative
Classic seminoma (dysgerminoma)	Sall4, OCT3/4, NANOG, D2-40, CD117, PLAP	panCK(−/+), CD30, Glypican3
Embryonal carcinoma	Sall4, OCT3/4, NANOG, CD30, SOX2, PLAP, panCK(+/−)	CD117, Glypican3, D2-40(−/+), AFP(−/+)
Yolk sac tumor	Sall4, PLAP(+/−), Glypican3, AFP(+/−), panCK(+/−)	OCT3/4, CD30, D2-40, NANOG
Choriocarcinoma	panCK, CD10, β-HCG, Glypican3(+/−), Sall4(+/−), PLAP(+/−)	OCT3/4, CD30, CD117, D2-40

−, <10 % of cases are positive; −/+, 10–50 % of cases are positive; +/−, 50–70 % of cases are positive; +, >70 of cases are positive
PanCK is positive in non-seminoma germ cell tumors but usually negative in seminoma/dysgerminoma

Identification of primary origin of a CUP would be of dramatic effects on disease staging, prognosis, and facilitate the choice of therapy for patients with these patients. Cytology is increasingly used in the investigation of CUP because in patients with advanced cancer, an FNA may be the only opportunity to obtain tissue or may be all that is necessary if surgery is not indicated. In addition, a rapid onsite evaluation can ensure obtaining adequate FNA material during the procedure. Pathologists should seek all available information before making a diagnosis.

A systemic algorithmic approach to identify primary origin of various malignant tumors has been addressed in the previous chapters. While new specific markers continue to emerge which will undoubtedly further improve the ability of pathologists to determine the origin of CUP, specific immunomarkers to detect some malignancies, such as cancers from gastroesophageal and pancreaticobiliary tumors, are still lacking. As a consequence, in a number of cases immunoperoxidase workup may only suggest a differential diagnosis rather than indicate a conclusive single diagnosis. Other tumors that often remain unclassifiable after an exhaustive use of immunostaining are the undifferentiated malignancies. In the current postgenomic era, molecular diagnostics using high-throughput methods such as microarrays have been explored to predict primary sites for patients with CUP and have shown promising results. However, molecular profiling is more complicated, expensive, and not accessible to most pathologists. The controversial issues on molecular testing are discussed in Chap. 7.

Prognostic and Predictive Markers in Cytology Practice

The predictive markers of breast cancer (i.e., ER, PR, and HER2) are usually tested via immunohistochemical staining on surgically resected or biopsy specimens of newly diagnosed primary carcinoma and require standardized processing conditions, as defined by ASCO/CAP guidelines. These markers are often requested by clinicians to test on cytologic samples of metastatic breast carcinoma to assess patients' eligibility for hormonal therapy and anti-HER2 therapy.

Cell block section is an ideal sample type for these tests, but it is not always available. Often, the marker study is requested retrospectively by a treating physician after a cytologic diagnosis has been completed when FNA smears are the only material available. In such situations, the existing smears that have been used for routine cytologic diagnosis may be used for ER and PR staining as long as technical validation has proven the reliability.

At MD Anderson, Papanicolaou-stained smears without destaining but with antigen retrieval are routinely used for ER and PR staining since an in-house validation in 2014 (Figs. 4.3 and 4.4). On the rare occasion in which tumor cells are present on a single smear but multiple tests are needed, a cell-transfer technique may be used. Of note, since these markers should be evaluated in the invasive component of the breast carcinoma and cytologic specimens cannot reliably discriminate invasive from in situ components, these tests should not be performed on primary breast carcinoma.

Unlike ER and PR, which are nuclear markers, HER2 is a membranous marker. Because the tumor cell membrane and intercellular relationship may be distorted during smearing, HER2 immunostaining should not be tested on smear preparation. FISH can be reliably used for testing HER2 status on direct smear (see Chap. 6). If cell block is available, HER2 can be evaluated using immunostaining technique, FISH, or other in situ hybridization method.

The stability of hormone receptor status and HER2 status during disease progression has long been of clinical interest. The common questions are whether the status of these receptors can be altered by chemotherapy or targeted therapy and whether retesting these markers in metastatic breast carcinoma is necessary. Several large studies at MD Anderson indicate that hormone receptor and HER2 status are generally stable during disease progression by comparing the status of the primary tumors (performed mostly on surgical tissue sections) with the corresponding metastatic tumors (performed mostly on FNA smears); intervening endocrine therapy, anti-HER2 therapy, chemotherapy, metastatic site (locoregional vs. distant), intervals between the two assays (<5 years vs. ≥5 years), and sample type of the metastatic carcinoma (direct smear vs. cell block vs. core needle biopsy) do not significantly affect the concordance of these markers between primary and paired metastatic carcinomas. Discordant status occurs only in a small proportion of patients, and the underlying mechanisms are multifactorial, including biologic evolution, intratumoral heterogeneity, technical (preanalytical and analytical) inconsistency, and interlaboratory and interobserver variability.

Other prognostic and predictive markers, such as Ki67 (to predict prognosis of neuroendocrine tumor or breast cancer), CD117 (to predict Gleevec response in gastrointestinal stromal tumor), CD38 (to predict adverse prognosis in small lymphocytic lymphoma/chronic lymphocytic leukemia (SLL/CLL), and P53, are infrequently tested on cytology samples; if needed, using cell block material is ideal.

Suggested Readings

1. Abbruzzese JL, Abbruzzese MC, Lenzi R, Hess KR, Raber MN. Analysis of a diagnostic strategy for patients with suspected tumors of unknown origin. J Clin Oncol. 1995;13:2094–103.
2. Chu P, Wu E, Weiss LM. Cytokeratin 7 and cytokeratin 20 expression in epithelial neoplasms: a survey of 435 cases. Mod Pathol. 2000; 13:962–72.
3. Chu PG, Weiss LM. Keratin expression in human tissues and neoplasms. Histopathology. 2002;40:403–39.
4. Clevenger J, Joseph C, Dawlett M, Guo M, Gong Y. Reliability of immunostaining using pan-melanoma cocktail, SOX10, and microphthalmia transcription factor in confirming a diagnosis of melanoma on fine-needle aspiration smears. Cancer Cytopathol. 2014;122:779–85.
5. Conner JR, Hornick JL. Metastatic carcinoma of unknown primary: diagnostic approach using immunohistochemistry. Adv Anat Pathol. 2015;22:149–67.
6. Ferguson J, Chamberlain P, Cramer HM, Wu HH. ER, PR, and Her2 immunocytochemistry on cell-transferred cytologic smears of primary and metastatic breast carcinomas: a comparison study with formalin-fixed cell blocks and surgical biopsies. Diagn Cytopathol. 2013;41:575–81.
7. Gong Y. Significance of biomarker discordance in breast cancer from the pathologist's perspective. Cancer Biomark. 2012;12:207–18.
8. Gong Y. Ancillary studies on neoplastic cytologic specimens. In: Nayar R, editor. Cytology in oncology. New York: Springer; 2013. p. 13–29.
9. Gong Y, Han EY, Guo M, Pusztai L, Sneige N. Stability of estrogen receptor status in breast carcinoma: a comparison between primary and metastatic tumors with regard to disease course and intervening systemic therapy. Cancer. 2011;117:705–13.
10. Gong Y, Joseph T, Sneige N. Validation of commonly used immunostains on cell-transferred cytologic specimens. Cancer. 2005;105:158–64.
11. Gong Y, Sun X, Michael CW, Attal S, Williamson BA, Bedrossian CW. Immunocytochemistry of serous effusion specimens: a comparison of ThinPrep vs cell block. Diagn Cytopathol. 2003;28:1–5.

12. Gong Y, Symmans WF, Krishnamurthy S, Patel S, Sneige N. Optimal fixation conditions for immunocytochemical analysis of estrogen receptor in cytologic specimens of breast carcinoma. Cancer. 2004;102:34–40.
13. Hornick JL. Novel uses of immunohistochemistry in the diagnosis and classification of soft tissue tumors. Mod Pathol. 2014;27 Suppl 1: S47–63.
14. Huo L, Gong Y, Guo M, Gilcrease MZ, Wu Y, Zhang H, Zhang J, Resetkova E, Hunt KK, Deavers MT. GATA-binding protein 3 enhances the utility of gross cystic disease fluid protein-15 and mammaglobin A in triple-negative breast cancer by immunohistochemistry. Histopathology. 2015;67:245–54.
15. Huo L, Zhang J, Gilcrease MZ, Gong Y, Wu Y, Zhang H, Resetkova E, Hunt KK, Deavers MT. Gross cystic disease fluid protein-15 and mammaglobin A expression determined by immunohistochemistry is of limited utility in triple-negative breast cancer. Histopathology. 2013;62:267–74.
16. Knoepp SM, Roh MH. Ancillary techniques on direct-smear aspirate slides: a significant evolution for cytopathology techniques. Cancer Cytopathol. 2013;121:120–8.
17. Lin F, Chen Z. Standardization of diagnostic immunohistochemistry: literature review and geisinger experience. Arch Pathol Lab Med. 2014;138:1564–77.
18. Lin F, Liu H. Unknown primary/undifferentiated neoplasms in surgical and cytologic specimens. In: Lin F, Prichard JW, Liu H, Wilkerson M, Schuerch C, editors. Handbook of practical immunohistochemistry: frequently asked questions 2011. New York: Springer; 2011. p. 55–83.
19. Lin F, Liu H. Immunohistochemistry in undifferentiated neoplasm/tumor of uncertain origin. Arch Pathol Lab Med. 2014;138:1583–610.
20. Lin G, Doyle LA. An update on the application of newly described immunohistochemical markers in soft tissue pathology. Arch Pathol Lab Med. 2015;139:106–21.
21. Liu H, Shi J, Prichard JW, Gong Y, Lin F. Immunohistochemical evaluation of GATA-3 expression in ER-negative breast carcinomas. Am J Clin Pathol. 2014;141:648–55.
22. Marshall AE, Cramer HM, Wu HH. The usefulness of the cell transfer technique for immunocytochemistry of fine-needle aspirates. Cancer Cytopathol. 2014;122:898–902.
23. Moore JG, To V, Patel SJ, Sneige N. HER-2/neu gene amplification in breast imprint cytology analyzed by fluorescence in situ hybridization: direct comparison with companion tissue sections. Diagn Cytopathol. 2000;23:299–302.
24. Niikura N, Liu J, Hayashi N, Mittendorf EA, Gong Y, Palla SL, Tokuda Y, Gonzalez-Angulo AM, Hortobagyi GN, Ueno NT. Loss of human epidermal growth factor receptor 2 (HER2) expression in metastatic sites of HER2-overexpressing primary breast tumors. J Clin Oncol. 2012;30:593–9.

25. Reuter VE, Argani P, Zhou M, Delahunt B. Members of the IIiDUPG: Best practices recommendations in the application of immunohistochemistry in the kidney tumors: report from the International Society of Urologic Pathology consensus conference. Am J Surg Pathol. 2014;38:e35–49.

26. Schmitt F, Barroca H. Role of ancillary studies in fine-needle aspiration from selected tumors. Cancer Cytopathol. 2012;120:145–60.

27. Ulbright TM, Tickoo SK, Berney DM, Srigley JR. Members of the IIiDUPG: Best practices recommendations in the application of immuno-histochemistry in testicular tumors: report from the International Society of Urological Pathology consensus conference. Am J Surg Pathol. 2014;38:e50–9.

28. Wilkerson ML, Lin F, Liu H, Cheng L. The application of immunohisto-chemical biomarkers in urologic surgical pathology. Arch Pathol Lab Med. 2014;138:1643–65.

29. Xiao C, Gong Y, Han EY, Gonzalez-Angulo AM, Sneige N. Stability of HER2-positive status in breast carcinoma: a comparison between primary and paired metastatic tumors with regard to the possible impact of intervening trastuzumab treatment. Ann Oncol. 2011;22:1547–53.

30. Zhang YH, Liu J, Dawlett M, Guo M, Sun X, Gong Y. The role of SOX11 immunostaining in confirming the diagnosis of mantle cell lymphoma on fine-needle aspiration samples. Cancer Cytopathol. 2014;122:892–7.

31. Zhao L, Guo M, Sneige N, Gong Y. Value of PAX8 and WT1 immunos-taining in confirming the ovarian origin of metastatic carcinoma in serous effusion specimens. Am J Clin Pathol. 2012;137:304–9.

32. Varadhachary GR, Raber MN. Cancer of unknown primary site. N Engl J Med. 2014;371:757–65.

Chapter 5
Flow Cytometric Immunophenotyping

Flow cytometric analysis is a powerful tool to determine the lineage, phenotype, and other characteristics of hematopoietic cells. It uses the principles of light scattering and light excitation and the emission of fluorochrome molecules to generate specific multiparameter data from particles and cells. It is a highly sensitive technique that can quantify the expression of eight or more colors/markers on a single cell and therefore enables the identification of aberrant cells within a complex cellular background.

With the increasing use of FNA, this technique has become a main ancillary test to evaluate lymphadenopathy and hematopoietic neoplasms in cytology practice, especially in view of the considerable overlap of cytologic features among some types of lymphomas and between low-grade lymphomas and reactive lymphoid hyperplasia. Although histologic evaluation is standardly required for a diagnosis of any type of lymphoma in a primary setting, cytologic evaluation of FNA samples is often performed in the setting of persistent or relapsed lymphoma, particularly for mature B-cell non-Hodgkin lymphomas. The cytologic features of FNA samples, in conjunction with immunophenotypic information, are usually sufficient for a diagnosis in this setting. The antibody panel selection and the interpretation of phenotypic data should be based on the cytologic features and clinical information. In a primary setting in which a lymphoma is clinically suspected, the panel should include key antibodies to cover the B-, T-, and NK-cell populations; In addition, a concurrent core needle biopsy should be obtained for histologic confirmation, subclassification,

© Springer International Publishing Switzerland 2016
Y. Gong, *Metastatic Neoplasms in Fine-Needle
Aspiration Cytology*, DOI 10.1007/978-3-319-23621-6_5

and grading. Sample handling and triage have been covered in Chap. 2 and Fig. 2.1. The immunostaining results of the main hematopoietic malignancies are listed in Table 4.10.

Interpretation Issues

Mature B-cell neoplasms account for more than 85 % of non-Hodgkin lymphomas and are the most commonly encountered hematopoietic neoplasms in cytology practice. Therefore, evaluating clonality by assessing immunoglobulin light chains (i.e., kappa and lambda light chains), together with CD19 and CD20 expression, is important to establish a B-cell neoplastic nature (Figs. 5.1 and 5.2).

In nonneoplastic conditions, the specimen comprises a mixture of T and B cells. In addition to CD19, CD20, and CD22, mature nonneoplastic B cells typically express polytypic surface immunoglobulin. B-cell lymphomas, however, express a single clonal light

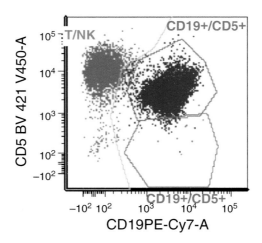

Fig. 5.1 Multicolor flow cytometric immunophenotyping on fine-needle aspiration sample (example 1): the histogram shows coexpression of CD19 and CD5, an important feature of mantle cell lymphoma

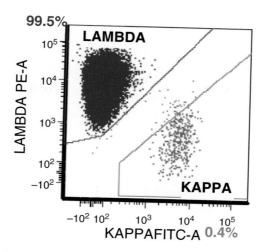

Fig. 5.2 Multicolor flow cytometric immunophenotyping on fine-needle aspiration sample (example 2): the histogram shows monotypic B-cell population with lambda light chain restriction

chain (also called light chain restriction), so the kappa-to-lambda ratio is either substantially increased or decreased due to a significant lambda excess. Ki67 immunostaining on cytospin preparation (Fig. 4.13) is often included in lymphoma workup to help tumor grading, to aid in the diagnosis of Burkitt lymphoma, or to confirm the blastoid nature of mantle cell lymphoma. The aberrant expression of some antigens in B-cell lymphomas may be of prognostic value. For example, CD38 expression in B-cell SLL/CLL is often associated with a more aggressive clinical course. Table 5.1 lists the key immunophenotypic and molecular features of mature B-cell neoplasms commonly encountered in cytology practice.

Although in most cases, the interpretation of flow cytometric data is quite straightforward, traps may be encountered. Correlation of flow cytometric data with clinical and cytologic findings and Ki67 staining is important. In rare cases, cytogenetic or molecular studies may also be needed. Interpreting a case solely on the basis of flow cytometric results may lead to an erroneous diagnosis. Negative findings do not necessarily indicate a benign process.

Table 5.1 Immunophenotypic and molecular features of mature B-cell neoplasms commonly encountered in cytology practice

Tumor type	Immunophenotype	Cytogenetic change
Burkit/atypical Burkitt lymphoma	CD45+, sIg+, CD79a+, CD19+, CD20+, CD10+, BCL6+, high Ki67 index (nearly 100 %)	Most common: t(8;14)(q24;q32); less common: t(2;8)(p12;q24) or t(8;22)(q24;q11)
	CD5−, CD23−	
Follicular lymphoma	CD45+, sIg+, CD79a+, CD19+, CD20+, CD10+ (occasionally CD10−), BCL6+	Most common: t(14;18)(q32;q21); rarely: t(2;8)(p11;q21) and t(18;22)(q21;q11)
	CD5−, CD23+/−	
Large B-cell lymphoma	CD45+, sIg+, cIg+ or Ig undetectable, CD79a+, CD19+, CD20+, high Ki67 index	t(14;18)(q32;q21)
	CD10−/+, BCL6−/+, CD5−/+	
Lymphoplasmacytic lymphoma	CD45+, sIg+, cIg+, CD79a+, CD19+/−, CD20+/−, CD38+, CD43+/−	
	CD10−, CD5−, CD23−	
Mantle cell lymphoma	CD45+, sIg+, CD79a+, CD19+, CD20+, CD5+, FMC7+, CD79a+, BCL1 (cyclin D1)+, SOX11+	t(11;14)(q13;q32)
	CD10−, CD23−	

Marginal zone lymphoma (splenic or nodal) and MALT lymphoma	CD45+, sIg+, CD79a+, CD19+, CD20+ CD10−, CD5−, CD23−, BCL6−	t(11;18)(q21;q21), t(14;18)(q32;q21), t(3;14)(p14.1;q32), trisomy 3, and trisomy 18 (more common in MALT lymphoma)
Plasma cell neoplasms	CD45+/−, cIg+, CD79a+, CD38+, CD138+, MUM1+, CD56+/− CD19−, CD20−, sIg−	t(11;14)(q13;q32)
Small lymphocytic lymphoma/chronic lymphocytic leukemia	CD45+, dim sIg+, CD79a+, CD19+/−, dim CD20+, dim CD22+, CD5+, CD23+, (CD38+, and ZAP70+: worse prognosis) CD10−, FMC7−	Trisomy 12, 13q14 deletion, 17p and 11q deletions

Abbreviations: *MALT* lymphoma mucosa-associated lymphoid tissue lymphoma, *Ig* immunoglobulin light chain, *sIg* surface Ig restriction, *cIg* cytoplasmic Ig restriction

- Immunoglobulin light chain restriction may not be detectable due to too few neoplastic cells, which may be masked by abundant benign lymphocytes, a situation often seen in T-cell-rich large B-cell lymphoma or a partially involved node. Gating on the large cell population may separate neoplastic large cells from the reactive lymphocytes. In the case of partial involvement by follicular lymphoma, typically CD10-positive B cells demonstrate light chain restriction, whereas CD10-negative B cells express polyclonal light chain consistent with a nonneoplastic nature. In difficult cases, immunoglobulin heavy-chain (IgH) rearrangement can be detected using molecular study (see Chap. 7).
- In some B-cell lymphomas, a flow cytometric immunophenotyping shows a polytypic B-cell population without light chain restriction owing to the aberrant loss of surface immunoglobulin expression (Fig. 5.3). Using different antibodies for each light

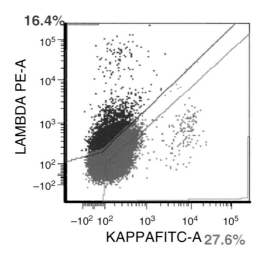

Fig. 5.3 Multicolor flow cytometric immunophenotyping on fine-needle aspiration sample (example 3): aberrant loss of surface immunoglobulin (kappa and lambda) expression in a follicular lymphoma, which leads to a "polytypic" appearance based on the histogram. Note, all the cells in this histogram are CD19 and/or CD20 expressed B cells. Histologic features and immunohistochemical workup of the lesion confirmed a diagnosis of follicular lymphoma

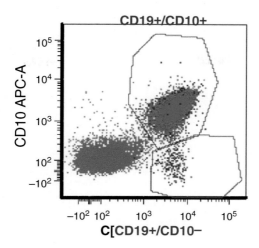

Fig. 5.4 Multicolor flow cytometric immunophenotyping on fine-needle aspiration sample (example 4): the histogram shows coexpression of CD19 and CD10, an important feature of B-cell lymphoma with follicular center cell origin

chain is important to verify true light chain loss or, in some cases, to overcome false negativity caused by an antibody issue.

- Since flow cytometric studies generally evaluate intact viable cells, poor cellular integrity, extensive fibrosis, and necrosis, which occur frequently in large B-cell lymphoma, may lead to a false-negative interpretation.
- Identical immunophenotypes may be seen in different types of lymphoma. For example, CD10-positive mature B-cell lymphomas include follicular lymphoma (Fig. 5.4), Burkitt lymphoma, and a subset of large B-cell lymphoma. On the basis of immunophenotypic data alone, the distinction among the three may be difficult. Clinical information (age or location of the lesion), cytologic features, Ki67 staining, and sometimes FISH studies will help the differential diagnosis (Table 5.1 and Chap. 6).
- Marginal zone lymphoma, mucosa-associated lymphoid tissue (MALT) lymphoma, CD10-negative follicular lymphoma, and lymphoplasmacytic lymphoma have similar immunophenotypes (i.e., monoclonal B cells with negative CD5 and CD10 expression).

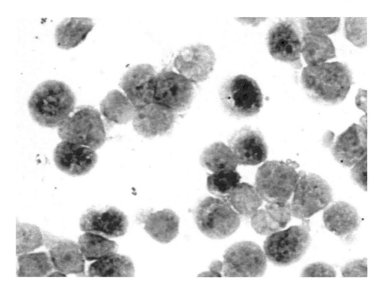

Fig. 5.5 An example of positive Epstein–Barr virus (EBV)-encoded small RNAs (EBER) by in situ hybridization on a cytospin to support a diagnosis of posttransplant lymphoproliferative disorder

- Large B-cell lymphoma may occasionally express CD5, resembling the phenotype of mantle cell lymphoma. Immunostaining for cyclin D1, SOX11 (Fig. 4.14), and FISH for t(11;14) (q13;q23) will help the differential diagnosis (Table 5.1).
- Posttransplant lymphoproliferative disorders resulting from immunosuppressive therapy in recipients of solid organ or bone marrow transplants are mostly Epstein–Barr virus related. These disorders range from reactive, polyclonal B-cell hyperplasia to those that are morphologically and genotypically indistinguishable from typical non-Hodgkin lymphomas. A positive finding of Epstein–Barr virus-encoded small RNAs (EBER), as determined via in situ hybridization, is supportive of its diagnosis (Fig. 5.5).
- The presence of a monoclonal B-cell population is not necessarily diagnostic for B-cell lymphoma. Some reactive conditions, such as Hashimoto thyroiditis and reactive lymphoid

hyperplasia in HIV-positive patients, may have small population of monotypic B cells. Caution should be taken not to over-interpret these conditions as lymphoma.

- Plasma cell neoplasms and some B-cell lymphomas are negative for surface light chain staining. In these cases, examination of cytoplasmic immunoglobulin light chains is the key to demonstrating clonality.

Compared to B-cell lymphomas, T-cell lymphomas generally have less predictable patterns of immunophenotypic aberrancy. T-cell lymphomas often show deletion or loss of one or more pan-T-cell markers (i.e., CD2, CD3, CD5, and CD7), which can be detected by flow cytometric immunophenotyping. In addition, T-cell lymphomas may demonstrate aberrant CD4 and CD8 patterns. In difficult cases, polymerase chain reaction can aid in the diagnosis by demonstrating clonal T-cell receptor gene rearrangements that are present in most T-cell lymphomas (see Chap. 7).

Suggested Readings

1. Caraway NP. Strategies to diagnose lymphoproliferative disorders by fine-needle aspiration by using ancillary studies. Cancer. 2005;105:432–42.
2. Chen HI, Akpolat I, Mody DR, Lopez-Terrada D, De Leon AP, Luo Y, Jorgensen J, Schwartz MR, Chang CC. Restricted kappa/lambda light chain ratio by flow cytometry in germinal center B cells in Hashimoto thyroiditis. Am J Clin Pathol. 2006;125:42–8.
3. Chen YH, Gong Y. Cytopathology in the diagnosis of lymphoma. In: Nayar R, editor. Cytology in oncology. New York: Springer; 2013. p. 211–40.
4. Gong Y. Ancillary studies on neoplastic cytologic specimens. In: Nayar R, editor. Cytology in oncology. New York: Springer; 2013. p. 13–29.
5. Gong Y, Caraway N, Gu J, Zaidi T, Fernandez R, Sun X, Huh YO, Katz RL. Evaluation of interphase fluorescence in situ hybridization for the t(14;18)(q32;q21) translocation in the diagnosis of follicular lymphoma on fine-needle aspirates: a comparison with flow cytometry immunophenotyping. Cancer. 2003;99:385–93.
6. Jorgensen JL. State of the art symposium: flow cytometry in the diagnosis of lymphoproliferative disorders by fine-needle aspiration. Cancer. 2005;105:443–51.
7. Katz RL RL. Cytologic diagnosis of leukemia and lymphoma. Values and limitations. Clin Lab Med. 1991;11:469–99.

8. Katz RL, Hirsch-Ginsberg C, Childs C, Dekmezian R, Fanning T, Ordonez N, Cabanillis F, Sneige N. The role of gene rearrangements for antigen receptors in the diagnosis of lymphoma obtained by fine-needle aspiration. A study of 63 cases with concomitant immunophenotyping. Am J Clin Pathol. 1991;96:479–90.
9. Kussick SJ, Kalnoski M, Braziel RM, Wood BL. Prominent clonal B-cell populations identified by flow cytometry in histologically reactive lymphoid proliferations. Am J Clin Pathol. 2004;121:464–72.
10. Verstovsek G, Chakraborty S, Ramzy I, Jorgensen JL. Large B-cell lymphomas: fine-needle aspiration plays an important role in initial diagnosis of cases which are falsely negative by flow cytometry. Diagn Cytopathol. 2002;27:282–5.
11. Wang J, Katz RL, Stewart J, Landon G, Guo M, Gong Y. Fine-needle aspiration diagnosis of lymphomas with signet ring cell features: potential pitfalls and solutions. Cancer Cytopathol. 2013;121:525–32.
12. Zhao X, Gong Y. Fine needle aspiration diagnosis of an early-onset post-transplant lymphoproliferative disorder. Diagn Cytopathol. 2011;39:788–90.
13. Zhao XF, Cherian S, Sargent R, Seethala R, Bonner H, Greenberg B, Bagg A. Expanded populations of surface membrane immunoglobulin light chain-negative B cells in lymph nodes are not always indicative of B-cell lymphoma. Am J Clin Pathol. 2005;124:143–50.
14. Zhang S, Gong Y. From cytomorphology to molecular pathology: maximizing the value of cytology of lymphoproliferative disorders and soft tissue tumors. Am J Clin Pathol. 2013;140:454–67.

Chapter 6
Cytogenetic Studies

Methodology of Cytogenetic Analysis

Cytogenetics refers to studying chromosomes in individual cells and their relationship to human disease. Abnormal cytogenetic findings can be found in the number and structure of the chromosomes, such as amplification, deletions, translocations, inversions, duplications, or isochromosomes. Conventional cytogenetic studies allow complete karyotype analysis using chromosome-banding techniques and detect most chromosome anomalies; however, it is a cumbersome and time-consuming procedure requiring adequate fresh tissue and special cell culture techniques in order to obtain an adequate number of proliferating cells. FISH, using fluorescently labeled probes, is currently more often used than conventional cytogenetic analysis because it is a relatively easy and fast technique to detect well-documented specific chromosomal abnormalities. It allows the localization of specific genes and DNA segments on specific chromosomes and may detect some abnormalities (e.g., microdeletions or duplications) that cannot be identified by conventional banding methods. FISH is particularly advantageous for FNA specimens because it can be tested on nondividing cells (so-called "interphase FISH") and only requires small number of cells. The drawback of FISH technique is that it requires knowledge of the specific loci involved in an aberration and is not informative to identify "unexpected" chromosome abnormalities.

© Springer International Publishing Switzerland 2016   163
Y. Gong, *Metastatic Neoplasms in Fine-Needle
Aspiration Cytology*, DOI 10.1007/978-3-319-23621-6_6

Sample Type of Cytogenetic Analysis

Cell block, direct smear (unstained or archived), cytospin preparation, and cellular touch imprint are all suitable for interphase
FISH. However, direct smear and cytospin preparation appear to
be superior to cell block sections because in this preparation gene
copy number can be enumerated on monolayered and whole tumor
cells with no nuclear truncation artifacts that is associated with
tissue section, thereby yielding a more accurate gene copy number.
FISH testing on previously stained archival smears has the advan-
tage of evaluating cytomorphologic features of the cells on the
same slides before FISH procedure. It is important to ensure that
the scoring should be performed on cells of interest instead of
background cells.

Common Applications of Cytogenetic Analysis

Identification of specific cytogenetic abnormalities has several
clinical implications:

1. Cytogenetic information can aid in more accurate diagnosis. For
   example, although cytologic features in conjunction with immunostaining or flow cytometric analysis are usually sufficient to
   make cytologic diagnosis, there are instances where identification of characteristic abnormalities at the chromosomal and/or
   molecular levels is necessary to arrive at a definitive cytologic
   diagnosis. For example, cytologic features of some mature
   B-cell lymphomas, such as follicular lymphoma, marginal zone
   lymphoma, or mantle cell lymphoma, can considerably overlap
   with one another as well as with those of reactive lymphoid
   hyperplasia. Some of these lymphomas, such as CD10-negative
   follicular lymphoma and marginal zone lymphoma, may share
   similar immunophenotypic features. A similar situation may be
   encountered in the cytologic diagnosis of sarcoma as well as
   small round blue cell tumors, a group of histogenetically different tumors that share morphologic features. Since lymphomas

and these solid tumors frequently carry nonrandom chromosomal aberrations (usually reciprocal chromosomal translocation), a cytogenetic analysis would be a powerful adjunct for the cytologic diagnosis. Tables 5.1 and 6.1 list the most common cytogenetic abnormality of these tumors (Fig. 6.1).

FISH can be used as a helpful diagnostic tool in salivary gland tumors because specific translocations are discovered in some tumors. For example, the t(12;15)(p13;q25) translocation resulting in ETV6–NTRK3 gene fusion is identified in >90 % of mammary analogue secretory carcinoma, the t(11;19) (q21;p13) translocation resulting in MECT1–MAML2 fusion gene in approximately 65 % of mucoepidermoid carcinoma, and t(6;9)(q22-23; p23-24) translocation resulting in MYB–NFIB fusion gene in approximately 50 % of adenoid cystic carcinoma.

Cytogenetic and FISH studies can also help the diagnosis of new variants of renal cell carcinoma, such as Xp11 translocation renal cell carcinoma and t(6;11) renal cell carcinoma (Table 4.17). Homozygous deletion of CDKN2A (P16) gene is the most common genetic abnormality in malignant mesotheliomas. The presence of such deletion, usually detected by FISH, favors a diagnosis of mesothelioma over reactive mesothelial hyperplasia.

2. Demonstration of characteristic chromosomal abnormalities may help in prognostic assessment. For example, the presence of the t(2;5) translocation in patients with anaplastic large cell lymphoma is associated with a favorable clinical outcome. In SLL/CLL, trisomy 12 and 11q and 17p deletions are associated with poor prognosis, whereas 13q14 deletion is a marker of good prognosis. The presence of t(11;19)(q21;p13) translocation or MECT1–MAML2 fusion transcripts in salivary mucoepidermoid carcinomas is associated with an indolent clinical course and is a favorable prognosticator.

3. Chromosomal abnormalities can be used to predict therapeutic response of some tumors. For example, positive HER2 status in breast carcinoma is a prerequisite for anti-HER2 (such as trastuzumab/Herceptin) therapy (Fig. 6.2). FISH testing for HER2 status is often performed on archival smears when cell

Table 6.1 Characteristic chromosomal abnormality in some soft tissue malignancies

Tumor type	Cytogenetic change	Fusion protein
Alveolar soft part sarcoma	t(X;17)(p11;q25)	ASPL–TFE3
Clear cell sarcoma/melanoma of soft parts	t(12;22)(q13;q12)	EWS–ATF1
	t(2;22)(q34;q12)	EWS–CREB1
Chondrosarcoma, extraskeletal myxoid	t(9;22)(q22;q12)	EWS–CHN
	t(9;17)(q22;q11)	RBP56–CHN
	t(9;15)(q22;q21)	TCF12–CHN
Dermatofibrosarcoma protuberans	t(17;22)(q21;q13)	COL1A1–PDGFB
DPSRCT	t(11;22)(p13;q12)	EWS–WT1
Endometrial stromal sarcoma	t(7;17)(p15;q21)	JAZF1–JJAZ1
Ewing sarcoma/PNET	t(11;22)(q24;q12)	EWS–FLI1
	t(21;22)(q22;q12)	EWS–ERG
	t(7;22)(p22;q12)	EWS–ETV1
	t(17;22)(q21;q12)	EWS–E1AF
	t(2;22)(q33;q12)	EWS–FEV
Inflammatory myofibroblastic tumor	Translocations at 2p23 involving ALK gene	TPM3–ALK
		TPM4–ALK
		CLTC–ALK
Liposarcoma, myxoid/round cell	t(12;16)(q13;p11)	FUS/TLS–CHOP
	t(12;22)(q13;q12)	EWS–CHOP

	Marker ring or giant chromosomes 12q13-15; amplification of MDM2 and CDK4	Amplification of MDM2 and CDK4
Liposarcoma, well differentiated		
PEComas	TFE3 rearrangement or amplification	TFE3
Rhabdomyosarcoma, alveolar	t(2;13)(q35;q14)	PAX3–FKHR
	t(1;13)(p36;q14)	PAX7–FKHR
Rhabdomyosarcoma, embryonal	Trisomies, 2q, 8, and 20	None
	Loss of heterozygosity at 11p15	none
Synovial sarcoma	t(X;18)(p11;q11)	SYT–SSX1
		SYT–SSX2
		SYT–SSX4
Wilms tumor	11p13 deletion/mutation	WT1
	11p15 mutation	
	Trisomy 12	

Abbreviations: *DPSCT* desmoplastic small round cell tumor, *PEComas* perivascular epithelioid cell neoplasms (including angiomyolipoma, clear cell sugar tumor, lymphangioleiomyomatosis), *PNET* primitive neuroectodermal tumor

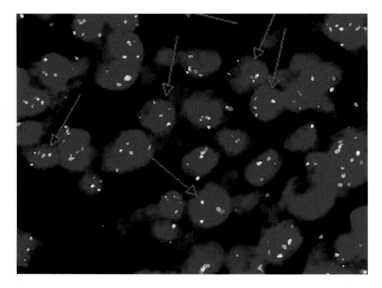

Fig. 6.1 An example of positive t(14;18) translocation detected by fluorescence in situ hybridization on a smear to confirm a diagnosis of follicular lymphoma

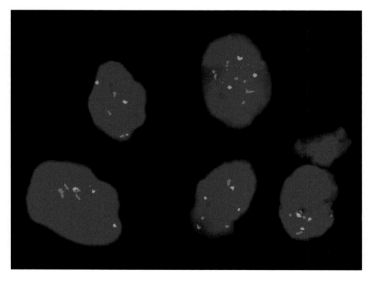

Fig. 6.2 An example of HER2 amplification by fluorescence in situ hybridization on a smear of a metastatic breast carcinoma

block tissue is not available. A t(2;5)(p23;q35) translocation causing gene fusion involving anaplastic lymphoma kinase (ALK) and echinoderm microtubule-associated protein-like 4 (EML4) can be found in about 4 % of patients with non-small cell lung carcinoma, which results in constitutive kinase activity that contributes to carcinogenesis. Positive EML4–ALK fusion detected by FISH is a prerequisite for using a small-molecule inhibitor of ALK (crizotinib/Xalkori) to treat patients with locally advanced or metastatic disease.

Suggested Readings

1. Beatty BG, Bryant R, Wang W, Ashikaga T, Gibson PC, Leiman G, Weaver DL. HER-2/neu detection in fine-needle aspirates of breast cancer: fluorescence in situ hybridization and immunocytochemical analysis. Am J Clin Pathol. 2004;122:246–55.
2. Caraway NP, Gu J, Lin P, Romaguera JE, Glassman A, Katz R. The utility of interphase fluorescence in situ hybridization for the detection of the translocation t(11;14)(q13;q32) in the diagnosis of mantle cell lymphoma on fine-needle aspiration specimens. Cancer. 2005;105:110–8.
3. Gong Y. Ancillary studies on neoplastic cytologic specimens. In: Nayar R, editor. Cytology in oncology. New York: Springer; 2013. p. 13–29.
4. Gong Y, Booser DJ, Sneige N. Comparison of HER-2 status determined by fluorescence in situ hybridization in primary and metastatic breast carcinoma. Cancer. 2005;103:1763–9.
5. Gong Y, Caraway N, Gu J, Zaidi T, Fernandez R, Sun X, Huh YO, Katz RL. Evaluation of interphase fluorescence in situ hybridization for the t(14;18)(q32;q21) translocation in the diagnosis of follicular lymphoma on fine-needle aspirates: a comparison with flow cytometry immunophenotyping. Cancer. 2003;99:385–93.
6. Klijanienko J, Pierron G, Sastre-Garau X, Theocharis S. Value of combined cytology and molecular information in the diagnosis of soft tissue tumors. Cancer Cytopathol. 2015;123:141–51.
7. Moore JG, To V, Patel SJ, Sneige N. HER-2/neu gene amplification in breast imprint cytology analyzed by fluorescence in situ hybridization: direct comparison with companion tissue sections. Diagn Cytopathol. 2000;23:299–302.
8. Okabe M, Miyabe S, Nagatsuka H, Terada A, Hanai N, Yokoi M, Shimozato K, Eimoto T, Nakamura S, Nagai N, Hasegawa Y, Inagaki H. MECT1-MAML2 fusion transcript defines a favorable subset of mucoepidermoid carcinoma. Clin Cancer Res. 2006;12:3902–7.

 9. Seethala RR, Dacic S, Cieply K, Kelly LM, Nikiforova MN. A reappraisal
    of the MECT1/MAML2 translocation in salivary mucoepidermoid carci-
    nomas. Am J Surg Pathol. 2010;34:1106–21.
10. Skalova A, Vanecek T, Sima R, Laco J, Weinreb I, Perez-Ordonez B,
    Starek I, Geierova M, Simpson RH, Passador-Santos F, Ryska A, Leivo I,
    Kinkor Z, Michal M. Mammary analogue secretory carcinoma of salivary
    glands, containing the ETV6-NTRK3 fusion gene: a hitherto undescribed
    salivary gland tumor entity. Am J Surg Pathol. 2010;34:599–608.
11. Shaw AT, Kim DW, Mehra R, Tan DS, Felip E, Chow LQ, Camidge DR,
    Vansteenkiste J, Sharma S, De Pas T, Riely GJ, Solomon BJ, Wolf J,
    Thomas M, Schuler M, Liu G, Santoro A, Lau YY, Goldwasser M, Boral
    AL, Engelman JA. Ceritinib in ALK-rearranged non-small-cell lung can-
    cer. N Engl J Med. 2014;370:1189–97.
12. Zhang S, Gong Y. From cytomorphology to molecular pathology: maxi-
    mizing the value of cytology of lymphoproliferative disorders and soft
    tissue tumors. Am J Clin Pathol. 2013;140:454–67.

Chapter 7
Molecular Studies

Genomic alterations are known to play an important role in cancer initiation and progression. Two main genetic events are considered to trigger cancer initiation: activation of oncogenes as a consequence of point mutation, amplification, or chromosomal translocation and inactivation of tumor suppressor genes due to chromosomal deletion, mutation, or epigenetic mechanisms. Molecular tests have been increasingly incorporated into pathology practice. Common applications include assisting pathology diagnosis, predicting prognosis and therapeutic response, and identifying patient's eligibility for targeted therapy.

Diagnostic Utility

Identification of primary origin of a metastatic disease is essential for an effective site-directed therapy. Although pathologic findings together with clinical and radiologic information and conventional ancillary tests, especially immunostaining, can effectively determine the primary origin in most cases (see Chap. 4), there are still some tumors in which their primary origins remain uncertain after extensive diagnostic workup. In recent years, molecular techniques have been explored in an effort to improve the detection of the tumor origin of CUPs. The techniques include gene expression profiling by detecting messenger RNA (mRNA) or microRNA using gene expression microarrays or real-time reverse

© Springer International Publishing Switzerland 2016
Y. Gong, *Metastatic Neoplasms in Fine-Needle
Aspiration Cytology*, DOI 10.1007/978-3-319-23621-6_7

transcription-polymerase chain reaction. These tests compare the gene expression profile in the CUPs to a defined gene set generated from various metastatic cancers with known origin to find the closest match. In addition to frozen tissue, small biopsy samples available as formalin-fixed and paraffin-embedded tissues and FNA samples are also suitable for the tests, with overall accuracy around 85 %. In some tumors in which tumor origin is doubtful or inconclusive based on immunostaining workup, molecular technologies provide additional clinically important information. Notably, one of the technologies (i.e., the Pathwork Tissue of Origin Test) has been extensively tested on cytology specimens and shows promising result.

However, controversy exists as to how much effort should be made in identifying the exact origin of a tumor, especially in the ear of next-generation sequencing (NGS), which is a powerful tool to detect actionable and driver mutations that may be targeted by specific therapeutic agents. Some clinicians believe that with known druggable targets and targeted therapies available, knowledge of a particular tumor origin may not be as critical as identifying the mutations that are amenable to molecular targeted therapies. However, gene expression profiling is expensive, is time consuming, and potentially exhausts tumor tissue. Low accuracy for poorly differentiated tumors is also a major concern because a genetic profile of such tumors may overlap. In most studies, the performance of gene expression profiling is generally similar to that of optimal immunoperoxidase workup. On the other hand, identifying the primary origin of a tumor still seems important for optimal treatment. For example, studies from MD Anderson group indicated that CUP patients with a gastrointestinal immunophenotype benefit from site-specific therapy that showed positive impact on survival. Furthermore, the meaning of a BRAF mutation in melanoma is very different from that in colon cancer or thyroid cancer. These findings compel a pathologist to identify primary origin of malignancy whenever possible.

Although the gene profiling approach is promising to improve the determination of primary origin of a CUP, additional studies remain to be done. Currently, gene expression profiling is not recommended as a part of the standard workup for CUPs. Therefore, using triple test to work up a CUP is still a fundamental practice. Immunostaining continues to retain its central role, with gene expression profiling serving as a potential adjunct in certain difficult cases. Meanwhile, discovering more novel site-specific immunomarkers with optimization and validation of their utility in small tissue samples like FNA materials is imperative.

Management of thyroid lesion largely depends on the FNA diagnosis. However, approximately 15–30 % of thyroid FNA diagnoses are indeterminate for malignancy. Multiple genetic mutations have been found to be associated with thyroid cancer. Molecular testing, ideally using fresh specimens, has been used as an adjunct to the cytologic diagnosis to increase the diagnostic certainty or avoid diagnostic thyroidectomy or may help in making decision on the extent of surgery in a patient with an indeterminate FNA diagnosis. A panel of molecular tests including *BRAF*, *RET*, *PAX8/PPAR gamma1*, and *RAS* helps to clarify some cases with indeterminate FNA diagnosis, with *BRAF* mutations being highly specific for thyroid carcinoma and RAS mutations being the least specific (Table 7.1). These genetic alterations are generally mutually exclusive of each other.

The presence of *BRAF* mutations or *RET/PTC* gene rearrangement is confirmatory to a diagnosis of papillary thyroid carcinoma. *RAS* mutations or *PAX8/PPAR gamma1* translocation are commonly associated with follicular thyroid carcinoma, a small subset of follicular variant of papillary thyroid carcinoma but can also be found in benign follicular adenomas. The other limitation of the molecular testing is that up to 30 % of thyroid cancers have no detectable mutation; therefore, management of the lesions that has an indeterminate FNA diagnosis and negative for the known molecular markers remains challenging.

Another approach to refine an indeterminate thyroid nodule is to use the Afirma gene expression classifier to identify whether the nodule has a benign gene expression pattern. Its result classifies nodules as "benign," "suspicious," or "non-diagnostic." The test has a generally high negative predictive value; however, it is also associated with a high false-positive rate, especially in Hurthle cell rich lesions.

Table 7.1 Average frequency of common molecular changes in thyroid tumors

Genetic alteration	PTC	FTC	PDCa	AC	FA	Comment
BRAF V600E mutations	45 % (classic>tall cell variant>follicular variant)		20 %	20 %		>90 % *BRAF* mutations
BRAF K601E mutations	3 % (follicular variant)	Rare			Rare	<10 % *BRAF* mutations
RET/PTC1 rearrangement (60–70 %)	15 % (classic type)					Often in adult patients who have radiation exposure
RET/PTC3 rearrangement (20–30 %)	5 % (solid variant)					Often in pediatric patients who have radiation exposure
N, H, KRAS mutations (*NRAS > HRAS, KRAS*)	15 % (mostly follicular variant)	45 %	30 %	50 %	30 %	
PAX8/PPAR Gamma rearrangement	2 %	35 %			7 %	Resulting from 2(2;3) (q13:p25) translocation
TP53			25 %	70 %		

Abbreviations: *PTC* papillary thyroid carcinoma, *FTC* follicular thyroid carcinoma, *PDCa* poorly differentiated carcinoma, *AC* anaplastic carcinoma, *FA* follicular adenoma

Molecular tests are also used for the diagnosis of lymphoma. Although diagnosis of most lymphomas can be reliably made based on conventional techniques such as immunostaining, flow cytometric immunophenotyping, and cytogenetic studies, a definitive diagnosis of a B-cell or T-cell neoplasms may be difficult in rare cases. Clonal B-cell or T-cell process may be confirmed only by molecular studies such as polymerase chain reaction which demonstrates immunoglobulin heavy-chain rearrangement for B-cell lymphoma and T-cell receptor gene rearrangement for T-cell lymphoma, respectively. Freshly FNA samples collected in cell-preservative medium are ideal for the tests.

Prognostic and Therapeutic Applications

The prognostic and predictive markers that might be tested in cyto-logic samples, such as ER, PR, HER2 status in breast cancer, *ALK* gene rearrangement in lung cancer, CD117 expression in gastrointestinal stromal tumor, Ki67 index in neuroendocrine and other tumors, and CD38 expression in B-cell SLL/CLL, have been addressed in Chaps. 4 and 5.

Detection of human papillomavirus (HPV) DNA in squamous carcinoma from the uterine cervix and oropharyngeal origins is not only helpful in the diagnosis but also of prognostic significance. Patients with HPV-positive oropharyngeal cancer tend to present with advanced-stage disease due to spread to the lymph nodes of the neck but paradoxically have a better prognosis than those with HPV-negative tumors. FNA materials of squamous carcinoma from head and neck sites, either cell block or direct smear, are often used for HPV testing using in situ hybridization, Hybrid Capture 2 or Third Wave (Cervista) Technologies.

Molecular revolution has led to an increasing effort to identify specific tumor mutations to enable adoption of genetically informed medicine for optimizing treatment and improving clinical outcome. In non-small cell lung cancer, detection of *EGFR* and *KRAS* mutation status on cytologic specimens is frequently requested by treating physicians to determine a patient's eligibility for anti-EGFR therapy (such as gefitinib/Iressa or erlotinib/Tarceva). Two classes of *EGFR* mutations, short deletions in exon 19 and the L858R point mutation in exon 21, are the most frequent mutations. The presence of *EGFR* mutations is associated with response to tyrosine kinase inhibitors. Major biomarkers *EGFR* (15–20 % in non-small cell lung cancer), *KRAS* (15–30 %), *ALK* (2–7 %), and *ROS-1* (1–2 %) are generally mutually exclusive. The tumors with *KRAS* mutations will not response to anti-EGFR therapy and likely have poor prognosis. NGS is a high-throughput sequencing technique that allows simultaneously identifying numerous DNA mutations that may have targeted therapies available.

To ensure a successful molecular testing, high quality of tumor sample is highly desirable. Cell block material or cells scraped from direct smears are suitable for the molecular studies with similar adequacy. Some studies show that smears are equivalent or slightly superior to cell block in mutational analysis. The efficacy of the molecular tests is affected to a great extent by the amount of tumor cells available for analysis. A total of approximately 10 ng of DNA is usually sufficient for NGS-targeted molecular profiling, depending on the testing platforms. A tumor percentage of >20 % is required for both smear and cell block preparations at MD Anderson. The number of slides required depends on the cellularity. For smears (either Diff-Quik stained or Papanicolaou stained), an average of 2 slides (range, 1–3) is usually required. For cell block, if the corresponding H&E section contains >300 tumor cells, an average of 5 unstained slides (range, 3–10) should be sufficient for NGS testing. In cases with <20 % tumor fraction, microdissection may be needed to enrich the tumor cells. Usually, if a molecular testing is anticipated, a pathologist should request more materials during rapid onsite evaluation, cut additional unstained slides upfront to avoid the loss of tissue due to repeatedly trimming of the cell block, judiciously select immunomarkers using systematic tired diagnostic approach, and consider dual or multiplex staining or transfer technique to save tissue. The goal is to maximize the cell availability for potential molecular studies, especially for a putative lung cancer.

Potential Future Application of Gene Expression Profiling

Gene expression profiling has been used to discover prognostic and drug response signatures for various tumor types and appears to be promising to facilitate personalized medicine because it allows for simultaneously measuring thousands of gene products from a single tumor sample. Gene signatures appear to provide more accurate prognostic and predictive information than any single gene measurement alone. In breast carcinoma, this technique has been used in identifying intrinsic subtypes, in developing prognostic signatures, such as the 70-gene signature (MammaPrint), and in exploring the gene signatures that predict tumor response to neoadjuvant chemotherapy, endocrine therapy, and other targeted therapies. FNA samples collected in RNA later can yield adequate amounts of total RNA in experienced hands.

With comprehensive microarray data available from nearly 500 patients, MD Anderson researchers found that the information of the important single markers such as hormone receptor and HER2 status can be reliably determined from the microarray data with a significant correlation between mRNA expression of ER and HER2 and the routinely determined status. These promising findings indicate that gene expression mircroarrays not only generate large and comprehensive gene expression data of breast cancer but also reliably measure ER and HER2; integration of the individual gene expression with multigene signatures generated from the same microarray data may potentially refine and improve predictive power for tumor response to targeted therapies and therefore optimize clinical decision-making and tailoring the therapeutic regimens on an individual basis.

In conclusion, with the rapid advent of sophisticated diagnostic technology and increased understanding of the molecular mechanisms of various tumors, the need to obtain diagnostic, prognostic, and predictive information from cytologic material continues to grow. Ancillary studies have played an important role in providing these information. Novel molecular technologies are emerging and will continue to improve the quality of patient care. The focus of treatment will shift from empiric therapies to more specific tailored regiments. As a pathologist, we not only need adoption and incorporation of the new techniques into routine practice but also should assume an active role in discovering novel site-specific markers and work closely with oncologists and radiologists to achieve the best patient care in the era of personalized medicine.

Suggested Readings

1. Aisner DL, Sams SB. The role of cytology specimens in molecular testing of solid tumors: techniques, limitations, and opportunities. Diagn Cytopathol. 2012;40:511–24.
2. Assersohn L, Gangi L, Zhao Y, Dowsett M, Simon R, Powles TJ, Liu ET. The feasibility of using fine needle aspiration from primary breast cancers for cDNA microarray analyses. Clin Cancer Res. 2002;8:794–801.
3. Billah S, Stewart J, Staerkel G, Chen S, Gong Y, Guo M. EGFR and KRAS mutations in lung carcinoma: molecular testing by using cytology specimens. Cancer Cytopathol. 2011;119:111–7.
4. Chowdhuri SR, Xi L, Pham TH, Hanson J, Rodriguez-Canales J, Berman A, Rajan A, Giaccone G, Emmert-Buck M, Raffeld M, Filie AC. EGFR and KRAS mutation analysis in cytologic samples of lung adenocarcinoma enabled by laser capture microdissection. Mod Pathol. 2012;25:548–55.
5. Dolled-Filhart MP, Rimm DL. Gene expression array analysis to determine tissue of origin of carcinoma of unknown primary: cutting edge or already obsolete? Cancer Cytopathol. 2013;121:129–35.
6. Gomberawalla A, Elaraj DM. How to use molecular testing results to guide surgery: a surgeon's perspective. Curr Opin Oncol. 2014;26:14–21.
7. Gong Y, Symmans WF, Pusztai L. Gene-expression microarrays provide new prognostic and predictive tests for breast cancer. Pharmacogenomics. 2007;8:1359–68.
8. Gong Y, Yan K, Lin F, Anderson K, Sotiriou C, Andre F, Holmes FA, Valero V, Booser D, Pippen Jr JE, Vukelja S, Gomez H, Mejia J, Barajas LJ, Hess KR, Sneige N, Hortobagyi GN, Pusztai L, Symmans WF. Determination of oestrogen-receptor status and ERBB2 status of breast carcinoma: a gene-expression profiling study. Lancet Oncol. 2007;8:203–11.
9. Greco FA, Lennington WJ, Spigel DR, Hainsworth JD. Molecular profiling diagnosis in unknown primary cancer: accuracy and ability to complement standard pathology. J Natl Cancer Inst. 2013;105:782–90.
10. Guo M, Khanna A, Dhillon J, Patel SJ, Feng J, Williams MD, Bell DM, Gong Y, Katz RL, Sturgis EM, Staerkel GA. Cervista HPV assays for fine-

needle aspiration specimens are a valid option for human papillomavirus testing in patients with oropharyngeal carcinoma. Cancer Cytopathol. 2014;122:96–103.

11. Hainsworth JD, Rubin MS, Spigel DR, Boccia RV, Raby S, Quinn R, Greco FA. Molecular gene expression profiling to predict the tissue of origin and direct site-specific therapy in patients with carcinoma of unknown primary site: a prospective trial of the Sarah Cannon research institute. J Clin Oncol. 2013;31:217–23.

12. Handorf CR, Kulkarni A, Grenert JP, Weiss LM, Rogers WM, Kim OS, Monzon FA, Halks-Miller M, Anderson GG, Walker MG, Pillai R, Henner WD. A multicenter study directly comparing the diagnostic accuracy of gene expression profiling and immunohistochemistry for primary site identification in metastatic tumors. Am J Surg Pathol. 2013;37:1067–75.

13. Hassell LA, Gillies EM, Dunn ST. Cytologic and molecular diagnosis of thyroid cancers: is it time for routine reflex testing? Cancer Cytopathol. 2012;120:7–17.

14. Kanagal-Shamanna R, Portier BP, Singh RR, Routbort MJ, Aldape KD, Handal BA, Rahimi H, Reddy NG, Barkoh BA, Mishra BM, Paladugu AV, Manekia JH, Kalhor N, Chowdhuri SR, Staerkel GA, Medeiros LJ, Luthra R, Patel KP. Next-generation sequencing-based multi-gene mutation profiling of solid tumors using fine needle aspiration samples: promises and challenges for routine clinical diagnostics. Mod Pathol. 2014;27:314–27.

15. Knoepp SM, Roh MH. Ancillary techniques on direct-smear aspirate slides: a significant evolution for cytopathology techniques. Cancer Cytopathol. 2013;121:120–8.

16. Nikiforov YE. Molecular diagnostics of thyroid tumors. Arch Pathol Lab Med. 2011;135:569–77.

17. Nikiforov YE. Molecular analysis of thyroid tumors. Mod Pathol. 2011;24 Suppl 2:S34–43.

18. Nikiforov YE, Nikiforova MN. Molecular genetics and diagnosis of thyroid cancer. Nat Rev Endocrinol. 2011;7:569–80.

19. Pusztai L, Ayers M, Stec J, Clark E, Hess K, Stivers D, Damokosh A, Sneige N, Buchholz TA, Esteva FJ, Arun B, Cristofanilli M, Booser D, Rosales M, Valero V, Adams C, Hortobagyi GN, Symmans WF. Gene expression profiles obtained from fine-needle aspirations of breast cancer reliably identify routine prognostic markers and reveal large-scale molecular differences between estrogen-negative and estrogen-positive tumors. Clin Cancer Res. 2003;9:2406–15.

20. Rosenfeld N, Aharonov R, Meiri E, Rosenwald S, Spector Y, Zepeniuk M, Benjamin H, Shabes N, Tabak S, Levy A, Lebanony D, Goren Y, Silberschein E, Targan N, Ben-Ari A, Gilad S, Sion-Vardy N, Tobar A, Feinmesser M, Kharenko O, Nativ O, Nass D, Perelman M, Yosepovich A, Shalmon B, Polak-Charcon S, Fridman E, Avniel A, Bentwich I, Bentwich Z, Cohen D, Chajut A, Barshack I. MicroRNAs accurately identify cancer tissue origin. Nat Biotechnol. 2008;26:462–9.

21. Rosenwald S, Gilad S, Benjamin S, Lebanony D, Dromi N, Faerman A, Benjamin H, Tamir R, Ezagouri M, Goren E, Barshack I, Nass D, Tobar A,

Feinmesser M, Rosenfeld N, Leizerman I, Ashkenazi K, Spector Y, Chajut A, Aharonov R. Validation of a microRNA-based qRT-PCR test for accurate identification of tumor tissue origin. Mod Pathol. 2010;23:814–23.

22. Stancel GA, Coffey D, Alvarez K, Halks-Miller M, Lal A, Mody D, Koen T, Fairley T, Monzon FA. Identification of tissue of origin in body fluid specimens using a gene expression microarray assay. Cancer Cytopathol. 2012;120:62–70.

23. Varadhachary G. New strategies for carcinoma of unknown primary: the role of tissue-of-origin molecular profiling. Clin Cancer Res. 2013;19:4027–33.

24. Varadhachary GR. Carcinoma of unknown primary: focused evaluation. J Natl Compr Cancer Netw. 2011;9:1406–12.

25. Varadhachary GR, Karanth S, Qiao W, Carlson HR, Raber MN, Hainsworth JD, Greco FA. Carcinoma of unknown primary with gastrointestinal profile: immunohistochemistry and survival data for this favorable subset. Int J Clin Oncol. 2014;19:479–84.

26. Varadhachary GR, Raber MN. Cancer of unknown primary site. N Engl J Med. 2014;371:757–65.

27. Weiss LM, Chu P, Schroeder BE, Singh V, Zhang Y, Erlander MG, Schnabel CA. Blinded comparator study of immunohistochemical analysis versus a 92-gene cancer classifier in the diagnosis of the primary site in metastatic tumors. J Mol Diagn. 2013;15:263–9.

28. Zhang MQ, El-Mofty SK, Davila RM. Detection of human papillomavirus-related squamous cell carcinoma cytologically and by in situ hybridization in fine-needle aspiration biopsies of cervical metastasis: a tool for identifying the site of an occult head and neck primary. Cancer. 2008;114:118–23.

Index

© Springer International Publishing Switzerland 2016
Y. Gong, *Metastatic Neoplasms in Fine-Needle
Aspiration Cytology*, DOI 10.1007/978-3-319-23621-6

Printed in the United States
By Bookmasters